MICHAEL O'DONNELL was a family doctor for twelve years before leaving clinical medicine to become an award-winning journalist and broadcaster. He presents the BBC television series *O'Donnell Investigates . . .*, is Chairman of Radio Four's *My Word!*, and for ten years has been a regular contributor to *Stop the Week*. In 1987 he enjoyed great success with his Radio Four series, *Relative Values*.

He has also written and presented television programmes about medicine and science in Britain and the United States and is a regular contributor to newspapers and magazines on both sides of the Atlantic.

Dr O'Donnell was editor of *World Medicine* for fifteen years and has been a member of the General Medical Council since 1971. His experience of business life includes eleven years as a director of a magazine publishing company and he is now a director of a film and video production company. For four years he has written a column on 'Executive Health' in each issue of *International Management* magazine.

He has published two novels, *The Devil's Prison* (1982), and *The Long Walk Home* (1988), and in 1986 came his first book about medicine: *Doctor! Doctor!, An Insider's Guide to the Games Doctors Play*.

DR MICHAEL O'DONNELL'S

EXECUTIVE HEALTH GUIDE

*How to succeed in business
without sacrificing your health*

LONDON
VICTOR GOLLANCZ LTD
1988

First published in Great Britain 1988
by Victor Gollancz Ltd,
14 Henrietta Street, London WC2E 8QJ

First published in Gollancz Paperbacks 1988

British Library Cataloguing in Publication Data
O'Donnell, Michael, *1928–*
    Dr Michael O'Donnell's executive health
    guide: how to succeed in business without
    sacrificing your health.
    1. Executives—Health programs
    I. Title
    613   RA776.5

    ISBN 0-575-04297-4
    ISBN 0-575-04262-1 Pbk

Photoset in Great Britain by
Rowland Phototypesetting Ltd, Bury St Edmunds, Suffolk
Printed in Finland by Werner Söderström Oy

For Frances, Lucy, and Jamie

Contents

Acknowledgements

The seed from which this book has grown was planted in my mind by a quiet American, Michael Johnson, who came to London in the winter of 1982 and invited me to write a regular column on 'executive health' in the magazine of which he had just become editor-in-chief.

Brave man that he is, he allowed me to take an untraditional look at an area of medicine which I felt was overburdened with stale dogma and old businesswives' tales and I'm happy to acknowledge that most of the ideas in this book were first floated in the column I still write in *International Management*. I've been encouraged to develop them further not just by Michael's enthusiasm but by the lively response that has come from the magazine's readers.

I'm also grateful to the many friends and patients who have given me permission to use their case histories to illustrate the arguments. They appear pseudonymously. The names used in the case histories are inventions, the stories are true.

What this Book is about

Most books about executive health try to sell you something: a new diet, exercise equipment, regular medical check-ups. This book tries to sell you nothing, apart from itself. It sketches an attitude to living that could make your work and play more enjoyable and your life less fraught with worry about illness and disease in yourself and in your family.

That attitude to living may be what people mean when they talk about health. One of the drawbacks to having been a doctor for over thirty years is that I have no clear idea of what health is. Certainly, I've seen patients with serious disabling diseases live what I thought were healthier lives than many businessmen and women who *knew* they were healthy because they had expensive X-rays to prove it, yet lived in unhappy conflict with everyone around them.

The track-suited persons who jog past my house clearly think health means physical fitness. Certainly there's no harm in jogging. Indeed there are lots of reasons for commending it. But I don't think physical fitness is the whole answer. The fallacy of equating it with health is exposed in the tale of the jogger who dropped dead while at his exercise. His running companion looked down at him proudly and said: 'What a way to go! In the peak of condition.'

For the purpose of this book I have assumed that health is closely akin to happiness. If we accept that notion, we don't, if we want to be 'healthy', have to become food faddists, obsessional joggers, or any other sort of health fanatic. Just by slightly altering the way we live, we can lower our chances of getting particularly nasty diseases like cancer and heart trouble and add not just years to our lives but years we will enjoy living.

This guide is not for people who think that health can be achieved only through suffering. It's more likely to appeal to businessmen and women who like to work hard and play hard but who do not want their zest for living to be impaired by unnecessary illness.

A HEALTHY STYLE OF WORKING

The Mythology of Stress

Coping with the myth of executive stress

Let's start with two simple truths:

- stress and tension are not an intrinsic part of any job but are generated by individuals

- the best way to avoid stress is to achieve some sort of harmony with the environment in which you work – advice which I admit is easier to enunciate than to follow

It's fashionable these days to talk about 'executive stress' as if it were a particular condition which occurs only at the top of the management tree, another status symbol to go with the leather-bound 'personalised' desk diary.

My experience, and that of other doctors, is that tension and anxiety are as common on the factory floor as they are in the executive suite and an industrial worker who spends his day doing a dull repetitive job may develop as serious symptoms of anxiety as the boss who scurries from meeting to meeting, from city to city, from country to country.

Another conceit of business is that if a decision involves a lot of money, it will be difficult to take and the taking of it will cause stress. The experience of doctors suggests that commoner sources of anxiety are small personal decisions which may seem easier to take but somehow remain untaken.

An even commoner cause of stress is uncertainty. The fear of redundancy is usually more stressful than the actual sack.

Yet while I don't believe there is a special élitist form of stress which affects only top level executives, I am interested in the ways in which the stress which can affect anybody can arise in a business setting.

An exact illustration of what I mean can be found in a film called 'Stress' made by Video Arts, a company justifiably renowned for its business training films. This film, with an accompanying booklet written by Dr Richard Lancaster, a consultant physician at St Mary's Hospital, London, is available for rent or for sale from Video Arts Ltd, Dumbarton House, 68 Oxford Street, London W1N 9LA. (Tel: 01-437 7104/0922 & 01-580 0652/0847.) It presents a day in the life of a manager under pressure not just from business problems – strikes at suppliers, demanding superiors, ambitious subordinates – but from domestic problems like his wife's migraine and his son's education.

It offers no simple solutions but gives viewers a chance to compare their own ways of business life with those of the central character, to see the steps he might have taken to ease the stress in his life, steps which they might take in theirs.

The film also avoids the trap of suggesting that all tension is a bad thing. It is tension, after all, that gives us the drive to be ambitious, to create, to succeed. A complete suppression of tension leads only to boredom.

The problem is that, while healthy work pressure can improve our performance, making us more efficient and our work more enjoyable, too much pressure can impair it.

The Efficiency/Tension Graph on the facing page carries two significant messages:

- the level of tension which produces maximum performance is close to that which causes deterioration

- when deterioration occurs, the decline is precipitate

Warning signs that the pressure is becoming too great include:

- an increase in alcohol, cigarette, or sleeping tablet consumption

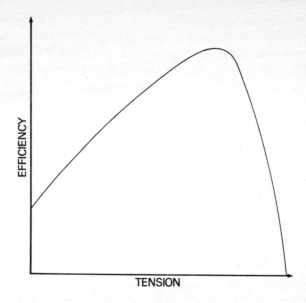

THE EFFICIENCY/TENSION RELATIONSHIP

- an inability to shake off a perpetual feeling of worry

- disturbed sleep

- a realisation that worry and fatigue are getting in the way of our doing our work as well as we used to

The anxiety which derives from unproductive tension is often accompanied by physical symptoms:

- certain sorts of headache (see page 27) and muscle ache

- dizzy spells and palpitations

- a constantly recurring feeling of tiredness which is difficult to shake off

If you recognise those symptoms in yourself, there are four practical steps you can take:

- **Establish your priorities**
  In the same way that making a list of things you have to do can sort out your day, so standing back and taking a cool look at the priorities in your life can help clear your mind of confusion, and you of stress.

- **Manage your time effectively**
  Trying to achieve more and more in less and less time impairs both your judgement and your creativity. Once you've established your priorities, why not make a list of tasks you have to do and allocate more time to the more important ones? A Filofax can be more than just a status symbol.

- **Delegate**
  Advice which I suspect has been repeated more than any other in business manuals, largely because it is so much easier to give than to follow. It may be true that you can do something quicker and better than any of your subordinates, but you will achieve greater efficiency if you spend your time on more valuable tasks.

- **Avoid isolation**
  Try to communicate with others. Too many managers call in their staff one at a time, listen, and then give instructions. If it's possible to get everybody together to share the problems, you'll be less likely to bottle them up. And bottled up problems are great provokers of unnecessary tension.

There's no need to wait until you suffer symptoms before you take those four practical steps. Take them now and you could prevent the symptoms from occurring.

And while you're at it, there are two other preventive moves you can make to keep yourself on the healthy side of the Efficiency/Tension Graph:

- **Away from your work, cultivate at least one activity which completely absorbs you**
  It can be a sport like golf or tennis. Or something less energetic like playing a musical instrument or running a club or society.

The secret of a 'laid back' tycoon

One of the most relaxed, easy-going men I know is a successful entrepreneur in a tough, competitive, and neurotic corner of the film industry.

In a play or film, his stereotype would be tense and restless, would guzzle tranquillisers, and would bustle through life radiating energy in every direction.

In real life, he is so 'laid back' that if he remains seated for too long, not just at home but in a plane or in the back of a car, or especially in a meeting, he drops off to sleep.

One of his party tricks, which he invariably performs at moments of business triumph or business disaster, is to gaze benignly at the excited or worried faces around him, give an exaggerated yawn, and say: 'I don't know that I can take the stress of this business much longer.'

He's made no conscious effort to insulate himself from the stress that's alleged to be an integral part of the film industry. But he does see that business in the context of a larger world. One of his better kept secrets is that he spent four years of his life in a concentration camp and, if pushed, will point out that to someone who stared death in the eye for a thousand days, any sort of day now is a bonus. He finds it hard to get steamed up about problems which may seem enormous when viewed from behind his desk but pall into insignificance when compared with some things he has seen men and women having to endure.

His success in business came, he says, because he established his priorities in life.

He could be right.

The only essential ingredient is that it should so absorb you that, when you engage in it, it commands your full attention and, for a refreshing hour or two, washes your mind clear of any lingering problems you brought home from the office.

Outside activities will bring you into contact not just with people who work in different businesses, or who have a different sort of working life. They will bring you into contact with some whose values have been fashioned by a wholly different style of living.

Don't dismiss them straight off. Listen to them. You may not be impressed by their attitudes or persuaded by their arguments but you may get some understanding of where your own style of living, and your own values, fit in the complex world in which we all struggle to survive.

- **Take one holiday lasting at least two weeks every year**
If you have an official holiday entitlement, take it. Don't say you'll make it up in odd days during the year. Apart from the fact that you won't – pressing work tends to get in the way – a couple of days off won't give your mind time to refresh itself.

If, when you go on holiday, you leave your phone number at the office, leave it with someone who will call you only when your advice *really* is indispensable – it rarely is. Never leave it with someone who will use it to bolster their insecurity or to duck out of responsibility.

Counting the cost

Sometimes, even though you've made all the right moves, and followed all the suggestions listed above, you may still find that every working day – not just an occasional run of days – has become an unhappy mixture of tension, dissatisfaction, indecision, and less than peak efficiency.

Don't just soldier on in a state of permanent disharmony with your working environment. That's a guaranteed route to damaging your health.

Analyse your problem in the way you analyse any problem that comes across your desk.

A useful technique is to take a couple of days off and, on your own or with someone who is very close to you, visit some quiet place where the ambience is as great a contrast as you can find to the hurly burly of your work. Then quietly and calmly set about analysing the cost of your job – to you, to your family, and to others who are important in your life.

When you make the analysis, you have to be ruthlessly honest with yourself. And that's not always easy, particularly if you spend your working days selling yourself to your customers or to your colleagues. It's difficult to drop the habit even when your only audience is yourself.

Yet, if you can achieve honesty in your appraisal, you'll find the exercise changes from being painful to being refreshing. Even for the most high powered of executives, confession *can* be good for the soul . . . and for the health.

When Jeremy Isaacs retired from the job of chief executive of television's Channel 4, he confessed to a group of colleagues that he had one bitter regret about his career, something that pained him all the more because it was then too late to repair the damage.

At one time he had worked seven days a week on two projects – as editor of *Panorama* and while making the series *World at War*. That work had won him great acclaim but he believed it had been earned at too high a cost to his family. 'Neither my wife nor my children saw enough of me in those years, or got enough of me when I staggered home exhausted.'

He offered this advice to his audience: 'Television is only television. No programme, however fulfilling, should keep us – need keep us – from those who love us best and need us most.'

His guilt may raise echoes in some who read this page. A lot of people earn success through obsessional involvement with their work. And though the obsession need not be painful – indeed, it is often highly enjoyable – the price it carries can be high. All of us should stand back occasionally and assess the price that we, and maybe others, are paying for our success. Often we will decide that it is worth it. Occasionally we may decide that it is not.

A common cause of debilitating tension is not just that that decision has never been made, but that it has never been faced. You will find one unexpected advantage can come from taking time off for self-analysis. The very business of looking closely at a problem often reveals simple practical solutions which up to that moment you were too busy to notice.

Anxiety: how understanding it can raise your efficiency

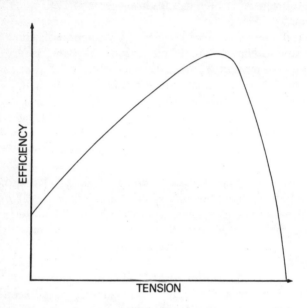

Take another look at the Efficiency/Tension Graph. If you allow your working tension to progress beyond the point of optimal performance, your efficiency will go into a precipitate decline. At that point any increased tension is not just unproductive but may affect your health.

It can do that by provoking one central symptom from which other symptoms flow. That central symptom is anxiety.

Anxiety is a great enemy of efficiency. Every businessman and woman will remember days on which their judgement and ability to make decisions were distorted by a worry which they hoped they had relegated to the back of their minds but which refused to stay there.

Anxiety is also exhausting. Coping with an unresolved worry can be as draining of energy as heavy physical exercise – without the compensating reward of a feeling of achievement.

I've already suggested how you can deal with – or, even better, prevent – the anxiety-provoking stresses that may be linked to your work. Another common source of anxiety in people who work under pressure is concern about their health.

They may suffer symptoms like headaches, indigestion, weariness, sleeplessness – often generated by the anxiety itself – which suggest they may be ill. Yet they don't really want to find out because they haven't the time to indulge in the luxury of illness, can't even afford the time to visit a doctor.

Ironically much of this anxiety is based on misunderstanding. Given an understanding of the nature of illness, people find that much of their anxiety evaporates. So a few minutes spent reading the next section may save you months of needless worry in the future.

It might even relieve you of anxiety that you suffer now.

Anxiety and illness

A patient of mine, wife of a high voltage marketing director, used to get an itchy rash on her left hand every two months. Usually it affected only one finger but sometimes it covered her whole hand. And it always started as a tiny patch around her wedding-ring.

When she saw a skin specialist, he suggested that her ring be tested for impurities to which she might be allergic. None were found and even when my patient didn't wear the ring, she still got the rash, starting at the point where the ring would have been.

As often happens when doctors are baffled, the patient came up with the answer. She noticed that the rash always started a few days before her husband was due to fly abroad on business. She herself was so terrified of flying that her family had once had to cancel a holiday when they arrived at the airport because she was too frightened to get on the plane. Discovering the link between her anxiety about her husband and her skin rash didn't cure the rash but gave it a name.

Skin specialists recognise 'wedding-ring dermatitis' as a rare affliction which sometimes occurs when a marriage is under strain or about to break up.

That rash was as dramatic an example as I know of the way that mind and body are irretrievably linked in disease.

These days most of us are prepared to accept that anxiety can cause headaches, or indigestion, even rashes, but the fact that it can cause a rash linked specifically to what is only a symbol may surprise even personnel directors who think they've seen everything.

Luckily, people responsible for managing large numbers of employees are less suspicious of psychology than they used to be, but it's extraordinary how many still refuse to prise themselves away from the cosy seventeenth century philosophy that mind and body are separate entities.

They recognise that anxiety produces physical symptoms, say in a student who has to dash repeatedly to the lavatory before an examination or in a subordinate who gets severe indigestion while preparing for a difficult meeting, but if a doctor suggests, no matter how delicately, that mental stress may be the cause of some of their own symptoms they assume the doctor is suggesting they are 'imagining' their troubles. And they resent it. They've got real physical symptoms so they want a real physical disease.

Yet the doctor isn't suggesting they're imagining anything. The pain of a tension headache is no less severe than that caused by a blow on the head from a mallet, the diarrhoea a student gets before an exam no less severe or uncomfortable than that produced by an infection. The symptoms are exactly the same: only the cause is different.

Some doctors suppress their own unease over conditions like the wedding-ring rash by calling them 'psychosomatic'. Yet 'psychosomatic', like 'wedding ring dermatitis', is only a label. And the labelling game is a dangerous one because it encourages us to think medicine is a matter of finding and applying 'cures' for 'diseases'. And that's not true.

True, people feel comfier with a named disease, but illness and disease are not synonyms. Every illness is unique, its nature determined not just by the assault from a disease or injury but by the mental and physical state of the individual who is assaulted.

This mysterious thing called illness

When I first met William Bennet of Sheerness, he was pregnant. At the age of seventy-nine, he found it a bit irksome but it was his thirtieth pregnancy and he had learned to live with the inconvenience.

Whenever one of his daughters or granddaughters was pregnant, his belly swelled and stayed swollen till the child was born. Oddly, he had never, as it were, come out in sympathy when his wife was pregnant.

Medical textbooks call Mr Bennet's condition 'couvade' but that is a label, not an explanation.

According to the dictionary couvade is a custom among primitive peoples by which a husband withdraws from the tribe, usually to an isolated hut, and 'feigns illness' during his wife's pregnancy. Mr Bennet withdrew from nothing and gave no impression of feigning anything, unless it was the cheerfulness with which he responded to his condition.

His experience is a dramatic illustration of the confusion that enters our minds when we assume that any abnormal physical state is an 'illness'.

Business managers often make this error. So do doctors.

Medical journals clearly regard Mr Bennet's experience as a medical phenomenon. Over the years they have reported a handful of cases similar to his but not one of the reports gives a clue as to what actually went on in Mr Bennet's abdomen.

But then, baffling the doctors is not as rare an accomplishment as some of them would have you believe . . .

Diseases can run such different courses in different people that they sometimes need different treatment, and a patient's determination to get better can sometimes have more influence on the course of an illness than high powered medical technology.

It's difficult to think of a more 'physical' illness than a broken leg yet, in a person who is fit and eager to get back to work, the bones will often knit more quickly than in one who is tired and depressed and who has little drive to get better.

Footballers can suffer painful injuries, even fractures, during a game and not notice them until the game is over and the excitement has drained out of them. The source of the pain is there all the time; what changes is the player's mental state. Similarly, the emotional stress of climbing the steps to the dentist's door or sitting in the dentist's waiting-room can suppress the pain of the toothache that caused the visit.

The fact that mental stress can cause illness doesn't mean that stress or tension are intrinsically bad. Without them most enterprises would grind to a halt.

Most of us, for most of the time, fit ourselves reasonably successfully into the pattern of life. Only when the pattern goes awry does the tension produce symptoms for us to take to the doctor.

Yet, even when we've delivered the symptoms to the doctor, there is no guarantee that he can do anything about them. I remember a patient who suddenly developed asthma in his late forties. We tested him for allergy to all sorts of dusts and pollens, but he reacted to none of them. Then his wife, a formidable and overpowering lady, died. He had no more asthma attacks. In a way he had been 'allergic' to his wife. If she hadn't died he might have got round to divorcing her, and that might have cured his asthma. But it also might have precipitated other troubles.

And therein lies a truth about illness that managers of large enterprises need to understand because of its effect not just on their employees but on themselves.

Illness is not always something dramatic that we switch on and doctors switch off. It's often an intermittent niggle that accompanies us through life and, like the lady with the 'wedding-ring dermatitis', we have to learn to live with it. She didn't try to get her husband to change his job because she knew he was happy doing it. She decided to put up with the rash and not let it get between her and enjoying life.

By that decision, her rash lost the status of a disease and became instead a nuisance that was only a minor part of a life she and her husband thoroughly enjoyed.

The symptoms that go with anxiety

Anxiety is probably the commonest cause of the symptoms which patients bring to their doctors. The anxiety may not always be recognised as such, even by the sufferer, and subconscious anxiety can cause a whole clutch of symptoms:

- **Tension headache**
  The commonest form of tension headache starts as a feeling of pressure, or sometimes just pain, on top of the head. This has a straightforward mechanical origin because anxiety or stress, call it which you will, can cause literal 'tension' in our muscles and make them tighten up.

  At the back of our heads and in our foreheads we have sheets of muscle which meet in a sheet of fibrous tissue which lies over the top of our skulls. When the tension in the muscles increases, they pull the fibrous sheet more tightly on to our heads and we may experience a feeling of pressure or of pain.

- **The original lump in the throat**
  This symptom of anxiety, occurs often – but not only – in people who fear, sometimes unconsciously, that they have cancer.

  They develop a lump in their throat which, when severe, seems to impede their swallowing.

  They don't imagine the lump. It exists all right and the mechanism which produces it is similar to that which produces tension headache because it consists of abnormal bulging of the throat muscles caused by increased muscular tension.

  The symptom, well recognised and described in medical textbooks, often – but again not only – occurs in people who have recently lost a friend or relative through cancer.

- **The anxious heart**
  There's a group of anxiety symptoms which occurs in people who have lost a friend or relative through heart disease. Medical text-books used to call it 'effort syndrome' – a few still do – and the symptoms include undue fatigue, shortness of

breath after even slight exertion, palpitations, and pain beneath the left breast – which, incidentally, is *not* where heart pain occurs.

Again the symptoms are not imagined. They really do occur and can be seriously debilitating. And it may take many investigations and a lot of sympathetic advice from a doctor to rid sufferers of their deep-down anxiety that they have serious heart disease.

Symptoms of anxiety such as those I've described don't occur only in the caricature 'worriers' who appear in cartoons or in the sort of people we regard as being 'riddled with anxiety'. They occur just as easily in seemingly tough extroverts.

To say that anxiety causes symptoms does not imply that the sufferers concoct the symptoms or that they are weak, inadequate people. In the world of business, they will include some of the most valuable, and most senior, individuals in a company.

Let me repeat – and the point is so important that it needs emphatic reiteration – the headaches caused by anxiety are just as real as those caused by a blow on the head, in the same way that the 'stomach upset' suffered by an executive on the eve of a vital meeting is just as real as the 'stomach upset' caused by an infection. The symptoms exist all right; it's just the cause that's different.

A lot of people are ashamed of admitting that anxiety could be a cause of their symptoms because they regard it as a sign of weakness. Anxiety, they think, is something they should overcome by 'pulling themselves together' and adopting more positive attitudes.

Yet though we tend to despise anxiety and to envy qualities which seem to deny it – like bravery and courage, which we attribute to ice-cool characters 'without a nerve in their bodies' – for most people, for most of the time, anxiety is something that is quite beyond their control.

We need to remind ourselves more often that true courage and true bravery are displayed not by those who are too stupid to know fear but by those who, plagued by anxiety, still manage to soldier on.

Mid-air consultation

He sat alongside me on an aircraft. Long before take-off, he had papers on his table and his fingers tapped a silent sonata on his pocket calculator. I too was busy reading but every time he interrupted his fingerwork he seemed to give me a shifty glance. By the time we were airborne, I was beginning to wonder whether I was paranoiac.

When the pre-lunch drinks arrived, he made his opening move. 'Seen you on the box. Talking about health. You'll be interested in the headaches I get from my blood pressure.'

The headaches, it seemed, were getting worse and he wondered what he could do about them. We still had 3,000 miles to travel and I wasn't going to escape so I asked how long he'd known his blood pressure was raised.

Eighteen months.

Had he had the headaches before then?

An occasional one, but not the same as these. Now they came more often and had a 'pounding' quality.

Had his doctor given his blood pressure a name?

Essential hypertension. (The fancy name doctors give to the commonest form of raised blood pressure for which we still don't know the cause.)

Last question. When his hypertension was diagnosed, did the doctor say how long he may have had it?

Probably for years. It had been found during a routine insurance examination.

So I passed on an aphorism I first heard as a medical student. 'Essential hypertension causes headaches only in patients who've been *told* they have raised blood pressure.'

I spent some time assuring him I wasn't suggesting he imagined his headaches. But they were more likely caused by anxiety than by his blood pressure. Once they started, anxiety generated by the fear that he might be about to have a stroke probably made them worse.

I think he accepted my assurances. When we'd finished eating, he put on his earphones and slept soundly through the movie, just like any normal business traveller. But that could have been the effect of the wine served with our lunch.

When to seek medical help

Soldiering on is not a good idea if your symptoms of anxiety persist too long. You should seek medical help if they:

- persist for more than a few days
- persist after the original cause has been removed
- arise when you can see no obvious cause
- start to interfere with your efficiency

The ways a doctor may help you include:

- helping you conduct the sort of analysis of the disharmony in your life described on pages 20–1
- teaching you relaxation exercises you can do to relieve the tension in your muscles
- using hypnosis or teaching you techniques of self-hypnosis with which you can treat yourself, perhaps using specially recorded tape cassettes
- giving you a short course of tranquillisers which will tide you over a difficult period or until you master an effective relaxation technique

Tranquillisers are effective dispellers of anxiety but doctors don't like to prescribe them indefinitely because people all too easily become dependent upon them. They are fine as a short term treatment which you can use to deal with crises or to buy you time to find a safer long term solution.

Understand Illness and be a Better Manager

Managing health and managing illness

One way to tackle the problems of illness is not just to treat the disease but to change the working environment of the victim. It's a technique which most of us don't use often enough. Yet it's a technique worth considering not just when valuable employees are ill but when we are ill ourselves.

There's nothing revolutionary about it. We all use it, albeit unconsciously, when the illness is mild or transient.

I've seen many a manager with the flu sitting up in bed, dosed to the eyeballs with aspirin, and working his way through a pile of paper which his secretary brought to his home from his office. But when the illness is serious or debilitating, a lot of companies seem to have a policy of 'pensioning off' employees who are ill rather than trying to adapt the job to accommodate the illness.

I would suggest, as an impertinent outsider, that that policy arises because too many companies, when they build their management structure, first define the executive jobs and then try to recruit people to fill them. Yet there's lots of evidence that spectacular success can be achieved by companies which first recruit talented people and then create jobs around them.

I've no doubt the 'job-filling' approach is administratively tidy and convenient but it leads too easily to the pensioning off approach to illness. And companies which routinely apply a pensioning off policy do seem, again to an outsider, to lose, quite unnecessarily, people whose training, experience, and under-standing of the business are valuable company assets.

Enlightened personnel departments are well aware of the technique of building jobs around valuable people and they use it often. What surprises me, as a doctor, is that the executives who manage those enlightened departments don't use it more often in their own lives.

One reason few of us do so is, I suspect, that most of us unconsciously assume that all people on this earth fall into two neat groups: those who are well and those who are ill.

For most of us, that vision of the world is reinforced by our experiences during the first two or three decades of our careers. We suffer an attack of influenza, or break an arm, or have our appendix out, and we see those illnesses as interruptions of our normal working life. We may have work brought to us in our hospital beds but that is a temporary expedient and real work starts again only when the accursed illness is out of the way.

As we grow older, however, we discover that health – which, as I keep reiterating on these pages, I like to think is more akin to happiness than to physical fitness – is not just a matter of the absence of illness but a much more positive entity. In my book, a man who is physically fit but who works in an environment with which he finds himself in permanent disharmony is not living a 'healthy' life.

And I find it sad that so many intelligent people who find themselves in that position think it is they who need treatment – be it with tranquillisers, psychotherapy, medical treatment for physical symptoms induced by the stress of frustration, or any fashionable nostrum of the moment – when really it is their working environment which needs 'treating'.

That is why I'm such an enthusiastic proponent of the technique of self-analysis described on pages 20–1. Any illness which disrupts the routine of our lives, even if it lasts only for a short time, offers another opportunity for self-analysis.

Indeed, it offers much more because not only can it give you a chance to review the value of the work you do and to wonder whether your life may need a change of direction; it also provides an excuse for making that change.

Illness can also remind us that being healthy means not just being mechanically sound in mind and body but involves our drawing satisfaction from the lives we lead, from the work we do, from using the skills and experience we have acquired.

Out of adversity came growth

When you make it to the top you sometimes get an extra perk. An unusual one came the way of a patient of mine some twenty years ago when he became the youngest member of the group board of a large British public company.

During his third board meeting, he developed symptoms of an impending heart attack and, though he didn't realise what was happening, his colleagues did.

The reason?

With only one exception, they had all suffered similar symptoms themselves.

Thanks largely to the medical histories of his fellow directors, my patient received the skilled medical help he needed – as it happened, just in time – and, when he returned from his convalescence, he was given a new assignment.

The incident had reminded the chairman just how many of his fellow directors had, like himself, had heart attacks and he conducted a discreet investigation into what extent the company was being deprived of valuable managers by illnesses which might have been induced by their work.

The findings so disturbed him that when my patient returned to work he was given the job of reorganising the group's management structure. The purpose was not to free senior jobs of all stress and tension – that would have been ridiculous. His brief was to devise a management structure which would reduce the sort of stress which leads to frustration yet not reduce, but encourage, the stresses which spur ambitious people to creative activity.

The reorganisation proved a mammoth task and I remember my patient telling me how he prevented himself from being confused by detail when faced by the more difficult decisions. At those moments, he would always go for the option that would make the manager's life more rewarding, not just financially, but as a job he or she would enjoy doing.

When I read the group's most recent annual report, I was reminded how that radical reorganisation sparked off spectacular success and growth which have been maintained ever since.

Reviewing your working life in those terms is a healthy exercise. Reviewing the lives of valuable employees in the same way is equally healthy – and profitable.

Mid-life crisis

Journalists who write about medicine in newspapers quickly discover that some topics provoke a dramatic increase in the number of readers' letters to the editor; not a mere doubling or a trebling but an inundation.

Sometimes the response comes as a surprise. A few years ago I suggested in a medical journal that many doctors who were good at their job had extracted most of their personal satisfaction from it by the time they were forty and they then started to grow bored.

The sackfuls of letters, nearly all from doctors claiming to be in the limbo I'd described, began to arrive within 48 hours and they kept on coming.

I've since returned to the subject many times in newspapers and magazines, on radio and television, and I've discovered that this yearning for a change of life is not confined to doctors but is shared by many a business executive who would never admit to its existence in public but is disturbed enough by it to seek solace in a confidential letter to a remote doctor who has done nothing more than describe it.

The 'I must change my job before I'm forty' syndrome seems most common among managers who work in specialised divisions like research but it is certainly not confined to them.

Most of the letters I receive make depressing reading. Some come from scientists who feel they had already done all the useful research they are likely to do, some from managers who have achieved most of the objectives they set themselves when they went into business. Nearly all ask me, as someone who seems to have had more than one career, where else, outside the mainstream of their profession, they might find work that would challenge their imaginations.

The saddest come from those whose relationship with their

work has followed a depressingly similar pattern: excitement, enthusiasm, and involvement in the early days, boredom entering, at first unnoticed, during their mid-thirties, then a recognition of the boredom followed by a growing feeling of imprisonment within a career which offers little flexibility and from which the only escape is a distant pension.

Many of my correspondents appear to reside in a cocoon: financially and socially comfortable but intellectually restless.

Successful companies, or at least those which haven't distanced themselves too far from their entrepreneurial origins, have a better track record than the professions or academic institutions in providing opportunities for flexible careers.

Yet as companies grow larger, 'career structures' grow less flexible. The impression I get from the victims is that many managements which try to provide their executives with regular opportunities for advancement still lay too great a stress on the neatness of a well-planned career, as if they were dealing with highly trained organisms and not with un-neat, quirky individuals.

That's why inflexible career structures remain a major cause of what is fashionably called 'the mid-life crisis'.

Inflexible career structures are also great promoters of mediocrity. Watching from the sidelines as a doctor, I've seen businesses not just lose but actively drive out some of their most valuable executives who were too individual, too rough around the edges, to fit the management pigeonholes they were expected to occupy.

The chances are that many who have read this far will already be painfully acquainted with the syndrome I've described. In too many companies – and professions – people who want to keep their minds alert and creative by changing the direction of their careers, are greeted with suspicion.

A 'career' becomes not a series of challenging opportunities but a prison.

Some people thrive on a lifetime commitment to one line of work but many commit themselves only because they're afraid to abandon a job that offers well-upholstered security to their families. No one would blame them for acting so prudently – it's

Escaping from the rut

For sixteen years Richard C was a respected and highly successful family doctor in a well-heeled corner of the Home Counties.

One afternoon he conjured up a vision of himself as an old man. He imagined his grandson sitting on his knee and asking 'Grandpa, what did you do with your life?'

And he heard himself reply: 'I went to medical school, qualified as a doctor, worked in a hospital for a year or two, then settled down as a family doctor in this pleasant town for forty years.'

The vision horrified him but, unlike many who suffer similar qualms in their mid-thirties or early forties, he decided not to brood but to act.

Three years later, after retaking examinations he thought he had left far behind him, he became physician to a school in the United States.

He says that uprooting himself, retraining himself, and searching for a different sort of job didn't demand much courage. It was a challenge and he enjoyed responding to it. His biggest worry was that he was being unfair to his family. Yet, once he'd started his new job, he and his family realised that the work and the anxiety had been worthwhile.

'I experienced a marvellous feeling of freedom. I'd proved it was possible to change the direction of my life. Passing the exams added to the pleasure because, by the time you reach forty, you wonder how rusty your brain has become.'

Yet the content of his new job was not much different from that of the job he left behind. His interest and enthusiasm were revitalised not so much by a change of work as by a change of environment. He also achieved another more subtle and more lasting change in his life.

He and his wife saw their move to the United States not as a once-and-for-all dramatic upheaval but as an episode in a continuum. After ten years in their new home, they would still have time for another adventure, with maybe a return to England where Richard could practise in yet another branch of medicine.

difficult to abandon habits that give an outward appearance of confidence yet conceal an underlying disenchantment – but such people are unlikely to provide the creative drive on which enterprises prosper.

Indeed, as advancing technology enables enlightened companies to delegate more and more routine tasks and decisions to machines, the management skill most in demand will be the creative versatility needed to invent and programme the machines. And that is a quality easily transferred from one sort of job to another. There has never been a better time for those who feel imprisoned by their careers to take the initiative they often dream about but never grasp.

I like the idea that life is a series of episodes in which a person's style of work can change to harmonise with changing social and intellectual demands. All the people I've met who have achieved that harmony find their work creative and rewarding.

Two management pitfalls

A simple misunderstanding of the nature of an illness or disability can lead managers into making decisions which harm not just their employees but their business.

This section deals with two medical conditions which are notorious for provoking bad management decisions.

Epilepsy: an illness that breeds prejudice

The setting was a small, high-powered management meeting held in a stately boardroom in the City of London. The half dozen participants, who had travelled from different countries, were conducting their business with professional calm when they suffered a dramatic interruption.

One of their number suddenly started to have an epileptic seizure.

The cool professionals suddenly became less cool. Indeed they grew distinctly panicky as they barked conflicting commands at one another. Their only point of unanimity was their need to find something they could force between the sufferer's teeth to stop him biting his tongue or choking on it. Then the chairman's secretary, a young woman who had been sitting quietly, invisible almost, in the corner, stepped forward.

She ordered her panicking elders to keep out of the way, gently guided the sick man to the part of the room that was least cluttered with furniture, eased his collapse to the floor, and stood by him for the thirty seconds the actual fit lasted, making no attempt to restrain him. And, while she waited, she asked her boss to ring for the company nurse.

She had dealt with the emergency in textbook fashion. The most helpful things a bystander can do for anyone suffering an epileptic seizure is try to prevent them from injuring themselves and to send for professional help.

There are also two things bystanders should refrain from doing. They should never try to hold down or restrain people who are having a fit. (Better to try and protect them from hard or sharp objects by shifting the objects that will move and padding those that won't with a coat or blanket.)

And – despite the popular belief – they should never try to force anything between the sufferer's teeth. That can do more damage than the sufferer is likely to do himself.

There are many forms of epilepsy. What they have in common is a sudden disturbance of the brain's electrical communication system which produces unconsciousness and the uncontrollable twitching and jerking of groups of muscles which we recognise as a fit. Brain cells communicate with one another by means of electrical impulses. In epilepsy, an electrical charge builds up in one group of brain cells and then suddenly discharges.

We don't really know what causes these electrical storms though we do know that two thirds of the people who suffer from epilepsy have no identifiable structural faults in their brains and that all of us are capable of producing a fit if our brains are subjected to intense repetitive stimulation.

Some people's brains can, for instance, be stimulated to the point of an electrical discharge by repetitive visual stimulation such as that produced by a strobe light, or even by the shadows of regularly planted poplar trees sweeping past a car window on a long straight road. Epilepsy seems to be an exaggeration of this normal response, as if the brain were 'oversensitive' to repetitive stimulation.

Drugs now exist to protect the brain against electrical over-activity and many epileptics rarely have a fit. Those who run any risk of having a seizure clearly have to avoid jobs that might, for example, involve driving, or climbing ladders, or handling dangerous machinery. But the risks must not be exaggerated. In the UK, for instance, epileptics who have not suffered a fit for at least three years while under treatment, can take out a driving licence.

Anti-epileptic drugs have also made it easier for sufferers to live normal lives and, if they wish, to keep their illness secret. That city manager who collapsed during the meeting was one who had chosen to do so.

When the drama in the office had subsided, the meeting's chairman found himself angered by the thought that a man had risen so high in the company without anyone knowing he was an epileptic. It took him some weeks to realise that the manager, like most people who suffer from the illness, was painfully aware of the prejudice it can arouse. Indeed, his decision to stay quiet could have been influenced by attitudes he'd seen fellow mana-gers take towards the illness, particularly when they were making decisions as employers.

Two hundred years ago, epilepsy was thought to be caused by possession by demons, and a whiff of the fear and superstition of those times seems to linger on. People who suffer from epilepsy still have to contend with irrational prejudice and, indeed, are often treated as if they were mentally impaired though they are likely to be as intelligent and imaginative as anybody else.

Recent surveys have shown that many epileptics lose their jobs when their condition becomes known, even when they have been doing work in which the rare chance that they *might* have a fit one day poses no hazard to themselves or those around them.

The same surveys show that the accident and sickness rates of people who suffer from epilepsy uncomplicated by other prob-lems are low. But such is the power of the myth – and survey after survey shows it is a myth – that epileptics have a poor work

---

Four recent victims of epilepsy prejudice

An export manager
who was 'eased out' of his £25,000 a year job after he had a
seizure at a diplomatic reception in Karachi

A fashion model
who ruined her career on the eve of signing a £100,000
five-year contract when she admitted 'as a matter of simple
honesty' to being a sufferer from epilepsy

A bride
whose husband left her after two months when a routine
medical check-up revealed that, though she had never
suffered an attack, she was potentially epileptic

A lollipop lady
aged sixty-eight, who lost her job, 'and my reason for
living', not because she had seizures but because old
medical records going back thirty years resurfaced and
showed she had once been diagnosed as having 'latent
epilepsy'

---

record, that many sufferers find that the only way to get a job is to
conceal their illness.

Concealment brings its own problems. Sometimes the illness is
revealed, as it was during that City meeting, in a disturbingly
dramatic way and a frightened manager may then respond by
dismissing the sufferer to protect himself and his colleagues from
another panicky experience.

I know the details of that boardroom meeting in the City of
London because the man who was chairing it described them to
me.

He has good reason to remember them.

Until that day he had always regarded his secretary as a quiet,
intelligent but rather dull person. Once she revealed the
personality she concealed behind her placid exterior, he took
more interest in her and, one year later, they were married.

Before the wedding she confessed a guilty secret. She too was an epileptic. He saw it as no barrier to their marriage but he still wonders whether, if he had known it earlier, he would ever have hired her as his secretary.

Discovering unseen talent

One winter evening a power failure blacked out a tall office block in the City of London. When five minutes later the emergency lighting also failed, the entire staff of a company which occupied two floors near the top of the building was led with unerring accuracy down an enclosed fire stairway by a junior member of the accounts department.

He apparently left the building by that stairway every evening because he found it easier to negotiate than the lifts. And he needed no emergency lighting because he was blind.

The company's chief executive, led by the hand down the dark staircase at the end of a line of equally helpless people, later discovered that the man who'd guided them was a gifted data analyst whose skill had escaped attention because his analyses were always written up in other people's reports. So one outcome of the power failure was that an unappreciated talent was recognised and rewarded.

I remembered the incident when I took part in a BBC radio programme for the blind. I was one of two sighted people who had to describe how we would respond in certain social circumstances involving blind or partially sighted people. Our answers were then discussed by a studio audience of blind and partially sighted people.

The main lesson I learned from the programme is one I'm sure I share with the people who were led down the stairway. Though we all know that blind people develop other faculties to compensate for their loss of sight, we often underestimate the extent to which they do so.

The blind chairman of our programme – working without notes – could instantly recall exactly who had said what during an hour's complex discussion. The junior accountant who led his colleagues down the dark stairway had to have figures read to him, unless they were printed in braille, but had developed a remarkable facility for analysing them.

Those images are worth remembering by all who employ, or work with, or have to manage, blind people.

Many companies waste the talents the blind have had to develop to overcome their handicap. Employers are always so conscious of the handicap itself that only rarely do they consider what talents are more likely to be found in blind than in sighted people, and how those talents might be exploited to their company's as well as their employee's advantage.

Many of us are not even all that good at understanding the needs of blind people who are colleagues or employees. A central lesson I learned from the BBC programme was that what blind people want most from those of us who seek to help them is honesty.

One of the questions we were asked was this: 'A blind neighbour asks you if you could read him a letter he's just received. When you glance at it, you see that it is anonymous, abusive, and obscene. Do you read it in full or do you skip some of the more insulting parts?'

My colleague on the panel opted for editing out the nastier bits and got short shrift from the blind audience. I said I would preface my reading with some remark like: 'This is an anonymous and abusive letter which, if it came to me, I would just glance at and throw into the waste bin. Do you want to hear it all?' But that also was too pussyfooting for the audience. They voted unanimously for having every word – including the four-letter ones – read to them exactly as they appeared on the page.

One of them pointed out that one of the most irritating things that can happen in their lives is someone offering to read a letter or a document and then paraphrasing it, giving the gist of a paragraph rather than the actual words. Blind people want to hear every word as printed, including the address and date printed at the top of a letter.

On reflection it is easy to understand why. They have to depend on others to supply them with data and, just like those of us who are sighted, they want to get those data in their raw form and make their own decisions about them.

Being honest with the blind means dealing with them as they are. They don't expect us to treat them as though they were normally sighted; that would be ridiculous. But they also don't want us to treat them as if they were handicapped in ways they are not. And they are not as embarrassed by their handicap as many of us fear.

None of our audience, for instance, would have minded being asked 'What sort of view do you take of that?' or 'Do you see it this way?' Indeed, some said they would delight in detecting the embarrassment in the speaker's voice as he realised what words he had used.

But they do have problems we often overlook. Their biggest worry when invited to a party, for instance, is how they are going to get home. If they fix up a lift beforehand or too early in the evening they may have to leave earlier than they want because their driver is leaving.

Another irritation is the fact they have no way of getting away early if they are bored. It's a freedom of choice that most of us take for granted. I certainly did until I spoke with a group of people to whom it was denied.

Blind people have a lot of useful information to give to their employers and their colleagues at work. Yet most of us, it seems, don't give them much chance to pass it on. We prefer to minister to the needs we *think* they have. That's a pity. We can't all rely on a power failure to give us a better understanding.

Travelling Healthily

Travelling in comfort

I started this book by admitting that I didn't know what health was though I hoped it might have something to do with happiness.

I also hope it may have something to do with comfort.

These days long distance business travel, with just a few golden exceptions, involves long distance air travel, and my observations at airports and in the air suggest that most people who travel frequently on business have already learned most of the wrinkles about travelling comfortably. The next section is therefore aimed mainly at the neophytes.

Air travel for beginners

The easiest way to diagnose the neophytes is by their clothing. Pin-striped suits or elegantly cut skirts and jackets look smarter in the departure lounge than they do in the arrival hall ten or twelve hours later. They're also not too comfortable if your destination is in the Far East and you arrive during the monsoon season.

I'm surprised – and depressed – by the number of business people I meet in tropical and subtropical countries who have left home without equipping themselves with appropriate clothing. I would have hoped that before they left home someone might have told them that the average Briton finds nylon shirts and underwear near to unbearable in hot and humid climates and that cotton is altogether more comfortable.

The best clothes for air travel are old, comfortable clothes. A few large pockets also come in handy particularly if at least one of them can be closed with a zip, and the second most desirable travelling companion is a friendly old sweater.

The first thing to do on boarding a plane is to get rid of coats and jackets, having first removed from them any valuables you want to keep close to you and anything you're likely to need during the flight, such as comb, spectacles, pen, or sweetener tablets. Then you can put on the old sweater you packed in your hand baggage.

You'll usually travel more comfortably if you take off your shoes and wear a pair of slippers. But remember your feet will swell during the flight. If you boarded the plane wearing tight shoes, you'd best not remove them or you may have difficulty getting them back on at the end of the journey. Better to travel in well-worn old shoes or loafers.

No experienced traveller worries too much about keeping up appearances while in the air. On most long distance flights the passengers in the first class cabin – which usually contains a high proportion of experienced business travellers – are invariably more scruffily dressed than those in the cabins behind. If you expect a formal welcome when you arrive, you can always nip into the lavatory on the plane or at the airport when you arrive and change into smarter clothes you've carried with you in a coat-hangered bag.

Another diagnostic feature of neophytes is their self-imposed tension which manifests itself as an urge to rush everywhere. Once you've checked in, the plane won't go without you – it's an inviolable security rule that all passengers who have checked in baggage must board the plane – and a senior British Airways doctor claims that self-induced stress in passengers who rush to the departure gate as soon as their flight is called is a well-known provoker of heart attacks.

If you travel a lot it's well worth joining one of the clubs run by most major airlines which allow you to sit in the calm of a private lounge until other passengers have boarded the plane. The lounges offer not just an ambience in which it is easy to work but insulate you from the tensions and anxieties of other travellers. Many years of travel under all sorts of conditions have convinced me that other people's tension is infectious.

Just as there's never any need to rush when you're on the ground, so there's no need to eat and drink everything that's served to you in the air.

On long hauls, the airlines sometimes have to serve meals to meet the needs of passengers who've boarded at intermediate stops. You're under no obligation to join in. If your body clock is registering 3 am, your digestive processes will have shut down for the night and anything you eat will linger for a long time in your stomach and bring you more pain than comfort.

Heavy drinking when your body clock registers an early hour of the morning will have the same effect as heavy drinking at the same hour on the ground. If you dislike the effect, you know how to prevent it . . . though you can deceive yourself by calling it jet lag.

The lowered barometric pressure in an aircraft cabin when maintained for a long time can accentuate the behaviour of the air which we all have within our bowels: the rumblings grow louder, the amount of wind seems to increase. In some people this apparent increase in 'wind' – it's not really an increase but an expansion of volume because of the decreased pressure – can provoke painful spasms of colic. It can also make tight clothes feel uncomfortable.

If you find 'the wind' troublesome, go easy on carbonated drinks – every airline carries gallons of still water – and on gas-producing foods. Some masochistic airlines still serve large helpings of beans.

The air conditioning systems used in aircraft can reduce the cabin humidity from the usual ground level of about 70 per cent to near 20 per cent. This drying of the air encourages much more water than usual to evaporate from your skin and through your lungs. To counter the dehydration you will suffer on a long flight you need to drink a lot of non-alcoholic fluid – three to four pints on a six hour flight.

Alcoholic drinks won't help. Indeed they'll make the dehydration worse because alcohol stimulates your kidneys to excrete more fluid than the drink contains. So if you are drinking alcohol on the plane, you will need to drink more than that three or four pints of water or soft drinks.

It's also a good idea on a long haul flight to get out of your seat occasionally and walk around the plane. Sitting still for long spells in a depressurised cabin can slow the blood flow through the veins of your legs. That's why your ankles swell and why some travellers, especially those who have varicose veins, later develop small patches of clotting in the veins of their legs. The clotting can be painful but is not dangerous. Walking around will speed up the blood flow, will reduce the risk of clotting, and also reduce the amount of swelling of your ankles. If you do have varicose veins, it's a sensible precaution to wear a light supporting stocking on long flights.

You can also stimulate the blood flow through your veins by clenching and relaxing your leg muscles while you're in your seat. A useful exercise is to raise your heel, press your toes hard against the ground, and encourage your leg to vibrate up and down by tightening and relaxing your calf and thigh muscles.

Lots of people find that exercising their leg muscles and doing similar exercises with their arms – pushing their hands hard together and contracting and relaxing arm and shoulder muscles – produces a refreshing feeling, as if they were washing away some of the physical staleness that comes with fatigue.

Some business trips involve carrying an increasing load of documents as the journey progresses so maybe it's not surprising that one of the commoner injuries suffered by business travellers is a pulled muscle or a strained shoulder joint caused by lugging around heavy suitcases.

Most of us on short trips try to carry all we need in our hand luggage in order to avoid that demoralising wait alongside the carousel in the arrival hall. If your hand baggage starts to grow burdensome, remember that you can unload some of those heavy documents on to the postal services or a courier. They're likely to be back at the office before you would have read them if you'd carried them yourself.

And if on a long journey you have to put one or two cases 'in the boot', it's worth using cases with built-in wheels. Airport corridors don't just *seem* to grow longer as we grow older (or wearier), they really are longer than they used to be.

Lastly, do remember there is more than one form of transport.

Because you have to travel to a country by air, it seems all too easy before you leave to book all your travel within the country on internal flights. Yet many countries still have first rate rail systems and a seat in a comfortable train makes a refreshing change from a seat in a depressurised cigar tube. A train also provides a more congenial working environment; you can spread your papers over more space and, even if you wish only to read, you can usually move away from noisy passengers rather than being compelled to sit alongside whomever the airline computer puts next to you.

Travelling by car

A hired car will allow you to break your journey when and where it suits you rather than the transport company. If you choose to travel long distances by car, pick the car in which you feel most comfortable – and that is not always the largest or the most expensive.

If you are travelling in your own or a hired car, a few simple precautions will ensure you arrive at your destination in a healthy – and this time it means efficient – state of mind.

If you have to launch straight into business action when you arrive, plan your route before you leave and pick not the shortest route but the one that is likely to provide least aggro. Allow time in your plan for breaks, not just for meals but for taking a brisk walk or even a short run. If you don't take a break you will arrive physically – and that also means mentally – stale.

Above all beware the trap that can be set for you by your own competitiveness – trying to get to your destination in the shortest possible time or to beat your previous record over the distance. If you're doing well against the clock, it's all too easy to stay behind the wheel and forgo those breaks you planned. You may get to your destination in record time but, when you do, much of the energy and drive you need to bring to your business will have been expended on the journey.

One advantage of car travel is that, if you have information or data recorded on tape cassettes, you can listen to it while you drive. If you're not in a business which deals with recorded information, record it for yourself. I know half a dozen actors who learn their lines that way. They read them into a tape recorder and then play them over and over on their way to their film location.

Travelling in comfort means using your imagination and not always choosing the most obvious route. Travelling by sea or river, for instance, may increase travelling time but it can refresh creative abilities exhausted by the breakneck dash too many of us feel we need to make if we are to be successful.

Coping with jet lag

Between a quarter and a third of travellers who have swept rapidly across several time zones have great difficulty adjusting to the new time, and about half of them have milder problems. I do mean several time zones – the one-hour difference which, for arcane reasons, British travellers still have to cope with when they visit mainland Europe will cause problems only in those with extravagant imaginations.

The commonest symptoms of jet lag are sleep disturbance, indigestion, hunger at odd hours, frequent urination, bouts of fatigue, diminished alertness, depression, anxiety, irritability, aggression and, sometimes, nausea and dizziness. Not all of these symptoms will occur in one sufferer and the severity of those which do occur will vary.

For business travellers, the most dangerous effect of jet lag is an impairment of performance – not just a diminution of physical strength and co-ordination, but slowed reflexes, a diminished capacity to learn and to remember, and a less acute sense of judgement.

These effects are particularly dangerous in someone conducting business because the sufferer also loses insight and does not appreciate the extent of the impairment. That is why many companies have a rule that no executive may sign documents on behalf of the company within 48 hours (some specify 72 hours) of arriving at a distant destination.

When travelling on business there are two strategies you can adopt to counter the effects of jet lag. If the trip is to be a short one, lasting for only two or three days, try when you arrive to stick as closely as you can to your home time and to schedule meetings and work sessions for what would be your peak times if you were at home.

The more senior you are, the more likely you are to have the muscle to fix timings to suit you. If you haven't the muscle, you can, in the days before you leave home, gradually shift your daily schedule towards that of your destination.

For longer stays at your destination, you need to adopt the second strategy. Now it becomes even more important to try and pre-adapt in the few days before you leave home by gradually shifting meal and sleep times to fit the new time zone. If your flight is a lengthy one, try to arrange a one-day stopover near the midpoint and, when you arrive at your working destination, adopt the new local time immediately.

During the first few days after your arrival, try to spend several hours out of doors: sunlight helps readjust your biological clock.

If you have the muscle to influence arrangements, try to start the trip with one or two not too strenuous days which will give you time to adapt to your new location before getting involved in more rigorous work. It will help if you avoid overeating and excessive use of alcohol while you're trying to readjust.

It's also a good idea to encourage your sleep pattern to re-establish itself and to counter the debilitating effects of jet lag insomnia by taking a short-acting sleeping tablet for the first few nights after your arrival. Most doctors prescribe a short-acting benzodiazepine but it's wise, before you leave home, to consult a doctor who knows you to make sure this sort of drug is suitable for you.

A lot of doctors will also advise you not to drink too much alcohol while you're in the plane, because many of the symptoms which travellers ascribe to jet lag are those of a hangover. Certainly you should try to counter the dehydrating effect of the dry air that's recirculated through the cabin by drinking lots of non-alcoholic fluids but, when it comes to alcohol, I rather like the attitude of one of my friends who told me: 'Whatever I do, I always feel bloody awful when I arrive, so I might as well have a pleasurable reason for feeling that way.'

Invisible hazards

It's no great secret that rapid air travel has led to rapid travel of diseases. Flu epidemics, for instance, sweep along more rapidly than they used to. Another effect of accelerated travel gets less attention. Because a businessman can work in an office in Europe one day and two days later may be doing the same job in the same sort of office in Africa or Asia, he can easily forget the threats the new environment may pose to his health.

He doesn't feel he has made an adventurous journey into dangerous territory. The people around him aren't all that different from the people at home. Sometimes their skin may be a different colour but they behave in much the same way as he does. They may well speak the same language, make the same sort of jokes, do the same sort of work, and face the same sort of problems. The environment in which most business people operate – offices, good hotels, restaurants – doesn't look or feel any less safe than the environment at home.

Small wonder that those who travel regularly can grow blasé about threats to health, fail to keep their jabs up to date, forget to take their anti-malarial tablets, and, above all, forget that their work abroad exposes them to illnesses that would not come their way at home.

Most British doctors learn little about tropical diseases at medical school and they can get caught out because their patients are not just travelling more but are growing more adventurous in their choice of destination. Recently a medical journal published the case history of an eighty-two-year-old grandmother who went on a round-the-world trip and caught malaria.

If you want to grab someone's attention about the effects of modern travel, just tell them a wider range of tropical diseases now exists in Northern Europe than can be found in any country in Africa. The statement is surprising until you analyse it. It creates the paradox by referring to the 'range' of diseases, not to the numbers of cases. European travellers returning from Africa may bring back different diseases from each country, whereas each country may have a lot of cases but a limited range of diseases.

Dr Alan Woodruff who is professor of medicine at the University of Juba in the Sudan, and was previously professor of tropical medicine at London University, has calculated that approximately one in ten people living in Britain is now exposed to tropical or subtropical diseases each year. If the time of possible exposure is expanded to two or three years, the proportion is much, much higher. And the people most at risk are not the tourists for whom a trip to the tropics may be a once-in-a-lifetime expedition but the business people for whom international travel is part of their working lives.

The explosive increase in international business travel has led most companies to set up administrative procedures to ensure that all employees who travel are given every protection that medical science can offer. American doctors have responded by creating a new medical speciality with an impressive new name. The entity that most of us used to describe as 'Travel Medicine' has now been transmogrified into 'Emporiatrics' – a word derived from *emporos*, the ancient Greek word for a traveller.

Experienced business travellers, if they are sensible, take a keen interest in emporiatrics and the true distinguishing mark of the professionals is that, if they are suddenly dispatched or summoned overseas, their protective inoculations will be up to date. If you wish to emulate them, which inoculations should you concentrate on?

Before you set out on any trip which may involve even just a brief stop in the tropics, ask your doctor about anti-malarial protection. In many countries it can be life-saving and I am appalled by the number of business travellers I meet in malarial areas who are quite unaware of the need for protective drugs.

Recently malaria has shown signs of resistance to some drugs. This resistance first appeared in Asia, possibly because of the quantity of the drugs taken by troops during the Vietnam war, but it has since spread to East Africa and if you visit certain

Infection	Do you need inoculation?	How long is inoculation effective?
Yellow Fever	Compulsory for visitors to parts of Africa and Central and South America. When not compulsory, still strongly advisable for visitors to those areas	1 injection produces protection that starts after 10 days and lasts 10 years
Typhoid and Paratyphoid	Essential for visitors to places where water supply may be contaminated. Typhoid can kill	2 injections, 10 to 28 days apart, give protection for 3 years
Cholera	Inoculation not especially important. Cholera is not the plague many people fear it is and is dangerous only if the dehydration it produces is not treated	2 injections, a minimum of 14 days apart, said to offer 6 months' protection, but are not wholly effective
Polio	You should be inoculated whether you travel or not, though travel puts you at greater risk	If not previously vaccinated, 3 monthly oral doses. A booster may be needed after 10 years. Check with your doctor
Tetanus	You should be inoculated whether you travel or not, though travel puts you at greater risk	2 injections with a booster every 5 years
Hepatitis	Advisable if visiting tropical or subtropical countries	One injection of gamma globulin protects for 3 to 6 months

Invisible imports

A chap I know, who wings his way round the world trying to sell industrial machinery to reluctant buyers, was recently laid low with flu. His temperature stayed up longer than it should and his GP grew puzzled.

Then the patient's boss visited him and gave the doctor the diagnosis.

The boss had lived for ten years in Africa and had seen more cases of malaria than had the English GP.

Travel was so much part of the machinery salesman's life that it never crossed his mind to tell his doctor he had recently spent a week in Indonesia.

He's not the only one.

A legal executive in a London solicitor's office was dismissed because of his repeated absences from work with bouts of vague abdominal pains. A psychiatrist diagnosed him as suffering from 'maternal dependency' but he recovered with amazing speed when he was given treatment for hookworms.

He had never told his doctor that he had taken a holiday in Africa.

countries you will be advised to take two different drugs to guard against the disease being resistant to just one.

The growing resistance of the malaria parasite to drugs has emphasised the need for that other protective measure against malaria – avoiding being bitten by a malarial mosquito.

The disease is carried by the female mosquito which most commonly emerges after the sun has gone down. So, when you're in a malarial area it's worth wearing clothes that cover as much of your skin as possible – high collars, long sleeves and long trousers (as opposed to shorts) after dark.

The past few years have seen the re-emergence of traditional anti-malarial devices like mosquito nets, repellent creams, and insecticide sprays, and the introduction of some new ones like plug-in heaters which, through the night, slowly convert a solid chemical tablet into mosquito-repelling fumes.

Patterns of other tropical diseases are also changing and, to get up-to-date information, you should consult a doctor before you leave; not any old doctor but one who really knows about foreign travel. He or she may not be an emporiatrician – I have yet to meet one – but try to find one who has access to the latest international data on diseases and on the health risks in the areas you will visit.

If you go to your own GP for advice, there's a useful hint you can pass on. Not many doctors know that the Hospital for Tropical Diseases in Liverpool always has a consultant on stand-by to answer queries from GPs about any of their patients who are travelling.

One thing you should never do is rely on books like this to prepare you for an overseas trip. The information I've listed is far from comprehensive and by the time you read it may well be out of date. Nor should you rely on your travel agent, nor even on your GP, unless he or she takes a special interest in the medical needs of travellers.

Airlines will give you more reliable information than travel agents, especially airlines like British Airways which have their own medical departments. And the doctors who can give you the most up-to-date advice are those who work at the Hospitals for Tropical Diseases in London and in Liverpool. (See below.) If you feel ill or run a fever soon after an overseas trip, don't assume it's the flu or a minor ailment. Consult a doctor . . . and don't forget to tell him where you've been.

Useful sources of information

- British Airways runs an Immunisation Unit which is also a rich source of practical advice. (Tel: 01-439 9584.)

- MASTA is the acronym of the Medical Advisory Service for Travellers, based at the London School of Hygiene and Tropical Medicine, and run by Dr Paul Clarke. The service maintains a regularly updated databank of health conditions in some 230 countries.

For a small fee (in 1987 it was £4.75), MASTA will supply basic health advice and an immunisation schedule for an overseas trip. For a larger fee (£9.50 in 1987) you get a guide to the health risks you are likely to run and advice on how to guard against them.

Once a traveller's personal health details have been fed to its computer, MASTA can produce further health briefs within one day. It runs a 24-hour telephone service and offers computer access to its data to companies with busy travel departments.

MASTA offers other useful services, including a health advice compendium for executives contemplating complex journeys or about to take up an expatriate posting, and can supply sterile medical equipment packs for use by travellers if they are involved in accidents or need emergency treatment in places where lack of sterile medical facilities could carry a risk of hepatitis or of AIDS.

MASTA can be contacted at the London School of Hygiene and Tropical Medicine, Keppel Street, London WC1E 7HT. (Tel: 01-631 4408.)

The commonest travellers' affliction

Most travellers have a tale to tell about the curse which struck their bowels when they visited some foreign part. The affliction is sometimes regarded more as a joke than a disease – though rarely at the time – and tends to have a different name depending on where the victim was struck down: Gyppy tummy, Montezuma's revenge, Delhi belly, The Mexican Two-step . . . I could fill half this page with the variations.

Diarrhoea is by far the commonest affliction suffered by international travellers. Two physicians who monitored 4,127 travellers passing through one European airport found that 36 per cent of them had had diarrhoea while abroad or immediately after returning home. That study also revealed that the most common sufferers are those least experienced in overseas conditions. But they are not the only ones.

In 1968, a one-day session of a medical conference in Tehran had to be abandoned because most of the doctors attending it had been stricken by severe diarrhoea. The subject of the session? Travellers' Diseases. And a US professor of medicine suggested in 1960 that American athletes lost their Olympic medals not on the running track but on the toilet seats of Rome.

More recently, the New York Philharmonic Orchestra was deprived of its entire string section during a tour of North Africa, and in 1985 one steamer-load of doctors who travelled down the Nile before attending a British Medical Association conference in Cairo saw less of Egyptian antiquities than of the inside of the steamer's lavatory.

Although diarrhoea may be a symptom of serious disease, and anyone who is seriously ill with it or in whom it persists for more than 24 hours should seek medical advice, the commonest forms of travellers' diarrhoea, though they often have a dramatic start, usually clear up quickly.

The most likely cause is an infection of the lining of the bowel by germs that enter the body in food or water, though doctors have long suspected that some cases may arise because the victim's intestine is unable to cope with a surfeit of unusual foods and drinks. This suspicion was strengthened when a team of research scientists investigated every case of diarrhoea occurring in a group of Europeans living temporarily in North Africa and found a causative germ in only 50 per cent of the sufferers.

What can you do to lower your chances of being struck down? There are a few simple precautions:

- don't eat large quantities of food to which your digestion is unaccustomed, particularly during the first few days after you arrive

- drink only boiled water. Water which emerges from an expensive tap or which is placed on the table in an elegant carafe may have come from a less elegant environment

- avoid iced drinks, unless you know for yourself that the ice was made from previously boiled water

- don't sample the local ice cream

- avoid uncooked food, particularly green salads. Be wary of raw seafood and undercooked meat. Indeed, eat only *recently* cooked food. It was a cold buffet that knocked out the doctors on the Nile steamer before the Cairo meeting

- remember you have no guarantee that dairy products, though they look wholesome, are uncontaminated

- never eat peeled fruit unless you have peeled it yourself

As an extra protection, some doctors recommend that their patients take a protective course of sulphonamide drugs while they are in infected areas, but these do not guarantee immunity. What should you do when the dreaded diarrhoea strikes?

- rest as much as you can

- stick to a light diet

- if you don't feel like eating, take fluids only

- if you can manage to swallow drinks which contain some salt – say a teaspoonful to a litre – you may prevent yourself from becoming too dehydrated

- take a 'bunging-up' remedy

The old notion that it was a bad idea to 'bung up' the diarrhoea in its early stages has proved to be a myth. There's now a range of effective 'stopper' drugs that doctors can prescribe. I usually rely on an old-fashioned one called codeine phosphate and your own doctor will be able to recommend one that should be suitable for you.

Anticipating trouble

When an overseas trip means spending time in out-of-the-way places, it's worth carrying a small medical kit to meet routine and emergency needs. Even if you don't have to use it, its psychological value is well worth the small amount of space it will take up in your baggage. Such a kit should include:

- first-aid dressings, now often available in sterile packs
- adhesive tape and scissors
- antiseptic cream and solution (or moist sterile 'wipes')
- antihistamine tablets (useful for allergy to insect bites and as mild sleeping tablets)
- an antibiotic prescribed by your doctor, for use only in the way and in the circumstances that he advises
- thermometer
- mild pain reliever: aspirin, paracetamol, ibuprofen
- hydrocortisone cream for skin rashes or insect stings
- antacid for indigestion
- diarrhoea 'bunging-up' medicine
- insect repellent
- sunscreen liquid or cream
- water sterilising tablets
- anti-fungal foot powder

You may need to expand this list to suit your individual needs. A nasal spray, for instance, is useful for people who find that pinching their nose and blowing out their cheeks as their plane descends does not always clear the Eustachian tube which runs from nose to ear.

If you are taking prescription medicines, carry them in your hand baggage, and you may save yourself a lot of problems at Customs and Immigration if the medicines are in their original containers and if the name on the label matches that in your passport.

Wise spectacle wearers always travel with a spare pair; even wiser ones also carry a copy of their last prescription.

If you fall ill while you're away, and you have access to a phone, it's worth calling your home doctor who knows your medical history. His or her advice is probably the best available to you, and the reassurance you get over the phone may be therapeutic.

No matter how skilful the local medical services may be, most of us find it hard to put complete trust in a doctor we've never seen before and who may have to communicate with us in his second language or in our second or third. If you do have to call in a local doctor, your own doctor will advise you on what to say to the local one or even speak with him or her on the phone.

If you have a chronic medical condition discuss its implications with your own doctor before you leave, and find out if there are any restrictions you should place on your activity or on your diet while you're away.

If you have a condition which needs special attention, like diabetes, heart disease, or a drug allergy, carry a note with you giving details of your medical history and try to find out before you leave what sort of medical services are available where you're going.

Medical insurance for business travellers has much improved over the past decade. Just one example of the sort of cover you can get now is that available to American Express cardmembers through Centurion Assistance. This insurance not only covers all your medical expenses (and those of your spouse and any children travelling with you) up to £1 million a year but will fly you home for medical treatment or fly out close relatives, an interpreter, or a personal doctor. Wherever you are in the world, all you have to do in the event of sudden illness or an accident is phone or telex a London number that is manned 24 hours a day and any medical help you need will be arranged. In 1987 the annual premium for this insurance was £85.

How to enjoy travel

Too many of us, when we travel, suffer from a condition I once defined as 'the Rolling Stone Syndrome'. Rolling Stoners gather no moss. We travel to new places, and, having looked without seeing and listened without hearing, roll home as uncontaminated as a highly polished billiard ball. One reason for our sad condition is that travel over long distances has become so easy. I do most of my travelling in the way of business and tend to nip into foreign cities, do my work, and nip back home, having cast little more than a token glance at the world around me.

So many of us do this nipping in and out that our habit has affected the architecture. Every major city in the world now has clusters of hotels which look as if they've been flung from the same giant concrete mixture and furnished from the same 'executive suite' catalogue. The same magazines are sold at each lobby news-stand, the same Muzak plays in each lift, and the same leathery prawns or even more leathery steak are flambéed in each restaurant.

Small wonder that persons who stay in these concrete palaces often forget where they are. The hotels usually lie at the centre of a cantonment of identical international airline offices, identical international car hire firms, identical travel agents, and identical expensive shops selling identical expensive goods by Gucci, Dior, or Dunhill. The absent-minded have to walk several metres, versts, or rods, poles, or perches to discover whether they're whooping it up in Düsseldorf or Leningrad or just spending an aberrant weekend in Birmingham.

Another contributing factor to the Rolling Stone syndrome is the habits that business travellers pick up from tourists, especially if they take an hour or two off to get away from the office ambience or to find out more about the country with which they are doing business.

Tourists now go to places not to pause and look around in wonder but to see things called 'sights' and to stare at stuff called 'scenery'. You can always identify a 'sight' because it is usually impossible to enjoy, and often impossible to see, because of its surrounding barrier of luxury coaches and crowds of oddly clad travellers gazing at history through Japanese viewfinders. Yet round the corner, untrod by foreign foot, may lie a shadowed alley that conveys more of the feeling of the place than half a hundred sets of concertinaed postcards.

Scenery is that stuff that you see from the window of your car or coach. It's not a place that man has lived in, or struggled to tame, or even a place where you should pause and let your imagination roam; it is stuff that has to be looked at, photographed, and written home about.

It is also something you can't afford to miss. Last autumn, I pulled my car off an Alpine road, into a lay-by enticingly labelled 'Vista'. As I stood on a rock, reluctant to move from surroundings with which I seemed to have achieved a magical harmony, another car pulled in alongside mine. A group of American businessmen got out, glanced cursorily about them, and then gazed confusedly at their map and guide book. Eventually one of them drifted over to me. 'It's truly magnificent up here,' he said, 'but I wonder if you could tell us which way we have to face to see the world-famous view.'

I apologise that these thoughts are so dyspeptic. I suspect I am trying to assuage my own guilt over the way I sometimes travel too hastily, taking for granted the privileges that are being afforded me. I also suspect it is my own guilt that depresses me when I see others who are alleged to be on holiday dashing from sight to sight with an urgency which denies them travel's greatest reward, that rekindling of the sense of discovery which we all knew as children and which we can still recapture if we are prepared to loiter in unfamiliar surroundings and give ourselves time to think and dream.

Travelling can, in short, be good for your health. And business travel need not be the chore that some people let it become. No matter how hectic your schedule you should try to carve some time out to spend not as a tourist but as a traveller.

A traveller, I suggest, is someone who looks beyond the sights listed in the tourist guides and seeks to understand the culture and the history of the people with whom he is doing business. And, just as you don't need to rush for the plane at the airport, so you don't need to rush at the places you visit.

Sex and the travelling businessman – and woman

You may think any advice I may offer on sex is surplus to requirements. A glance along the shelves of lobby bookshops in international hotels which cater for itinerant executives would suggest the market is near to saturation.

Most of those books, however, seem to be training manuals in sexual acrobatics or tourist guides to local attractions – with telephone numbers – which Baedeker overlooked.

I have good reason for thinking some businessmen and women would like a different kind of information.

Doctors like me, whom most people meet not in a formal consultation in a surgery or hospital but in a pub or club or non-medical office, attract a particular sort of question. People often manoeuvre us into a quiet corner and ask us questions they find it difficult to put to their own doctors – who may be long-time acquaintances – and much easier to put to a relative stranger who knows nothing of their home or their business.

Ten years ago most of the questions I was asked about sex were about sexual drive and sexual performance. Today the commonest questions are about sexually transmitted disease (STD).

The change in style of question began when herpes first appeared and accelerated with the appearance of AIDS. The threat of AIDS has now eroded some prudish public attitudes towards sexually transmitted diseases and reliable information about them is much easier to find.

Anyone who seeks a comprehensive account of them, their symptoms and their treatment should acquire a slim yet splendid book, *Sexually Transmitted Diseases: the Facts* (Oxford University Press) written by Dr David Barlow, a consultant at St Thomas's Hospital in London, who set out to produce a textbook for doctors and nurses but expresses himself in such clear prose that what he has to say can easily be understood by everybody.

He also offers friendly advice which is neither censorious nor condescending and even injects some humour into what need not be an unremittingly doleful subject.

Prevention is better – and often easier – than cure

In the current epidemic not just of AIDS but of other STD the 'travelling salesman', butt of so many sexual jokes, is at special risk. The jokes raise a laugh because they're based on a reality which most of us recognise – the itinerant businessman or woman in a hotel room, alone in the evenings, and far from home. The

Whatever happened to VD?

The coining of the phrase 'sexually transmitted disease' and substituting the abbreviation STD for VD sounds like an attempt to find a modern euphemism for an earthier historical entity. In truth the phrase venereal disease was abandoned because many countries had defined it legally and the definition was too narrow for the range of conditions treated in modern clinics. Certainly the change of name has coincided with a change of attitude towards treatment.

When I was a medical student in London in the early 1950s, the only public information about VD was that given in stilted official notices displayed in public lavatories, and the VD clinics in most hospitals – usually called 'special departments' – were housed in shabbier premises than those inhabited by more respectable specialities. True, they offered a confidential service but a person needed courage not just to go for treatment but even to inquire where the clinic was.

The spirit of those times is evoked for me by the tale of the music hall baritone who one evening after performing at a West End theatre arrived at the 'special department' at the old Charing Cross Hospital, dressed in tails, white tie, top hat, and white gloves. With a charming smile he told the receptionist: 'I have come in answer to your advertisement in the gentlemen's lavatory in Leicester Square.'

Few patients then could match that bravado; patients now don't have to try because today's clinics are easier to find and the nurses and doctors who work in them treat their patients with a kindly and uncensorious efficiency.

publishers of the 'local guides' on the hotel news-stands know that they have a ready audience.

The travelling executive can make two self-defensive moves against STD: one easy, the other not so easy.

The first derives from the simple mathematical truth that every time you take a new sexual partner you run the risk of getting a sexually transmitted infection, and that risk is multiplied by the number of people with whom your new partner has had recent sexual encounters.

An occasional woman with whom a travelling salesman has a one night stand in a distant city – or an occasional man with whom a travelling saleswoman has a similar encounter – *may* have led a wholly chaste life up to that moment but you'd have to be an intransigent self-deceiver to believe that such a circumstance was the rule rather than the exception.

So the simplest and most logical precaution anyone can take against STD is to avoid casual sexual relationships. But because logic rarely plays a part in sexual behaviour I regard that as the not-so-easy option.

The easier one used to be a matter of contraception but has now become a matter of protection. Infection in both men and women would be much reduced if, during casual sexual encounters, the man always used a condom.

The idea of a protective device is not new. James Boswell in his *London Journal*, written in 1763, described how in a casual sexual encounter he 'copulated free from danger, being safely sheathed' and used a memorable phrase to describe his discovery of the condom: 'For the first time did I engage in armour.'

For years before the outbreak of AIDS doctors had been advising men and women about the wisdom of using a condom when having intercourse with someone likely to have had as varied a sexual experience as they were attempting to have themselves.

The AIDS epidemic has now transmogrified that advice into a deadly warning. It also reminds us that modern medical technology does not have the answer to everything. We still need to remember the old soldier's maxim 'If you can't be good, be careful.'

Today's travelling executives, whose appetites are just the same as the eighteenth-century contemporaries of James Boswell, still have to rely on the same method of protecting themselves.

EXECUTIVE AFFLICTIONS

Most people, if asked to nominate the illnesses most likely to be suffered by business executives, would nominate those caused by stress.

As we have already seen (page 15), they would be wrong. Executives are no more prone to stress disease than anybody else.

To find what medical problems really do afflict managers, I enlisted the help of six British GPs who practise in suburban areas heavily populated by business commuters.

For three years they kept a record of the problems brought to them by their business executive patients – not necessarily the serious illnesses but the medical problems which the doctors judged were interfering with their patients' efficiency and their performance at work.

The conditions that topped that list form the content of this chapter. I don't include the figures of occurrence – the study was too small to be laden with statistical significance – but the order in which the afflictions appear – with the most common coming first – closely corresponds with the frequency they appeared in the GPs' diaries.

General Afflictions

Coping with a bad back

A few years ago I was summoned to the presence of one of Britain's captains of industry and, at the appointed hour, entered a palatial but empty office. As I perched on the edge of a chair, a deep voice, coming as if from heaven, filled the room.

'Is that you O'Donnell?'

Before I could reply, it boomed again.

'I'm over here behind the desk.'

I peeped beyond the massive desk and saw a tall distinguished man, immaculate in pin-striped suit, stretched on his back on the Aubusson carpet.

'One of your fellow quacks makes me do this,' he said. 'Twenty minutes every day, after lunch.'

For the next ten minutes we forgot the purpose of my visit and swapped experiences and helpful hints with the enthusiasm that back sufferers invariably muster when they discover one another.

I'm a fully paid-up member of the bad back club. My trouble started when, as an adolescent, I 'slipped a disc'. It would be nice to claim that the injury occurred before a full house at Twickenham or when I was serving to win championship point at Wimbledon but an essential characteristic of a 'bad back' is its mundaneness. Just as it allows its sufferers to earn little sympathy and much ridicule as they try to cope with it, so it allows little glory be won in its acquisition.

Mine first struck when I was perched on one foot and lazily manoeuvring a sock over the other. I fell backwards on to my bed and had to stay there for the following week immobilised by fear of the agonising girdle that embraced me whenever I tried to move. For ten years, I tried every form of treatment, orthodox and unorthodox. Then it dawned on me that, for many people, a 'bad back' is not so much an illness as a way of life.

Some people run a special risk – those, for instance, who are tall and who work at desks – but we've all been destined to suffer backache since the day our ancestors started walking around on their hind legs.

I'm sure if an engineer were to redesign the human body, he would put the main support, the bony spine, not at the back of the trunk but up the middle like a tent pole. Then its muscular 'guy ropes' could run at a wider angle and make it more stable.

Until a few more billion years of evolution move our spines into a more sensible place, those of us who are prone to backache will continue to learn the painful lesson that our comfort depends less on treatment than on prevention. That's why our lives become an endless quest after even better ways of protecting our backs and why we revel in exchanges of helpful hints such as that which occurred twixt me and the man on the Aubusson.

Positive action

- the first time severe backache occurs it must be medically investigated and treated. So must milder but continuing backache that lasts for more than a few days.

- once you've got medical assurance that no serious disease is causing your backache, you're in the hunt for effective relief.

  If your doctor seems unable to help you, ask around. You'll find fellow sufferers only too eager to tell you who 'sorted out' their back.

  But remember that a 'bad back' is one of the most individual of complaints. Treatment that helps one sufferer does not necessarily help another.

- when it comes to choosing between surgeon, physiotherapist, osteopath or chiropractor, you will discover that the world is divided into two distinct groups: those who can help your back and those who can't. If you find someone who can help your back, stick with them, whatever their title.

No matter how effective the treatment you eventually track down, most back pain sufferers end up with a niggly sort of problem which occasionally lays them low with acute pain and occasionally causes bouts of less severe pain which restrict movement and tend to make the sufferer irritable and short tempered.

Most of us can prevent those episodes if we teach ourselves to protect our spines from unnecessary strain. These days I get an episode of back trouble about once every four years (instead of once every four months) and it always occurs after an incident in which I've neglected the 'Dos and Don'ts'.

The 'Dos and Don'ts'

The most important 'Do' concerns posture: the need for us always to try reach our full height when standing. If you can face unpretty sights, stand naked in front of a bathroom mirror and then consciously let your body sag. The shock of what you see may persuade you never to do it when you're clothed.

- if you have to stand a lot at work, 'standing tall' protects your back and is much less tiring than slouching

- try not to stand with your weight mainly on one leg. If you can't break the habit, try to ensure you don't always favour the same leg

- if you have to sit for a long time, support the small of your back with a cushion or a roll

- interrupt long spells of sitting – on long journeys, for instance – by occasionally standing and stretching backwards to extend your spine

- always try to arch your back and tighten up your stomach muscles before you cough or sneeze

- sleep on a hard bed. Your mattress should be firm and should be placed on a firm base. (In emergencies, put the mattress on the floor.) The ideal base has no springs. If yours has, put a board – ¾ inch chipboard is best – between the base and the mattress to prevent it from sagging under you

- if you have to lift something heavy, always keep your back straight, the weight close to your body, both feet firmly planted on the ground in not too narrow a stance, and bend at the knees. The main lifting power should come from the muscles in your thighs working on your hips and knees, with your back remaining a rigid prop. Even better, don't lift heavy things. Get a mechanical device – or someone else – to lift them for you

- never, but never, lift anything with your spine twisted

- if your luggage is heavy, instead of one large suitcase, carry two small ones. The balance will keep your spine straight

- do not jerk or twist even when lifting quite light loads like bags of shopping, and try always to spread loads equally between both hands

- don't reach up to get things from a high shelf. Stand on a stool

- keep your back upright when you're sitting. Don't bend over your desk. Sit up straight and, if necessary, raise the work surface

- if you have to do something close to the ground – gardening, changing a plug – don't bend but get down on your knees or lie on your stomach or on your side

- buy a car with a driver's seat that supports the arch in your back and, if your present seat doesn't provide that support, slip a cushion between it and your lower back, or fit one of the seat frames designed to give proper support to your back

- if you have to spend a lot of your time sitting at a desk, try one of the backless chairs on which you perch in what looks like, but isn't, a semi-kneeling position. The good ones are surprisingly comfortable and the original Balans 'alternative sitting' chairs remain the best. Some of the cheaper imitations will protect your back but may also give you painful knees. Balans chairs don't do that

- the need to keep your spine in a safe position persists when work is over and you leave the office. Don't sag or slump in an armchair or a poolside 'lounger'

- try to relax your back for a spell each day. A good way is to lie on your back on the floor with eyes closed and a small pillow under your head. Keep your tongue gently against the roof of your mouth and deliberately relax each group of muscles, working up the body: feet, calves, thighs, bottom, stomach, chest, hands, arms, neck, jaw, face, eyelids. If, after doing that, you try to turn your eyes, still closed, to 'look inwards', you'll find you clear your mind of distractions, and after ten minutes, you'll feel enormously refreshed

- exercises to strengthen your back can also help but are best learned from demonstration by an expert or from an illustrated manual*

The healthy approach to coping with a bad back is to learn to live with it. Most back sufferers build the 'Dos and Don'ts' into their daily routine and adapt them to their style of work. Once upon a time writing at my desk was the commonest source of my backache but now I can perch on my Balans chair and tap away at my word processor for eight or more hours without getting one warning twinge from back or knees.

Indeed the chair has proved such an effective deterrent that my office now harbours a second one of different design in which I can sit and read or lie back and relax while keeping my vertebrae in safe alignment.

Back sufferers are better catered for than they used to be.

---

* The manual I'd recommend is *The Back: Relief from Pain*, a slim volume in the Positive Health Guide series (Macdonald Optima) which illustrates some useful exercises simply and clearly. It is also packed with commonsense advice by Dr Alan Stoddard who knows a lot not just about the human spine but about us back pain sufferers.

Furniture designers are at least becoming aware of our needs and it's worth shopping around for a chair or two in which you can relax comfortably and safely.

I've become an addicted visitor to The Back Store (324a King Street, Hammersmith, London W6 0RF, tel: 01-741 5022), the nearest thing I know to a back sufferers' Aladdin's cave. It is crammed not just with furniture but with all sorts of devices designed to help us sufferers cope with our affliction. And it is staffed by folk who really do understand our bizarre needs.

Dyspeptic status symbol

Whatever happened to that old time executive status symbol the duodenal ulcer? Not too long ago an ulcer was regarded as some sort of business battle honour, as prized a possession as a key to the executive washroom.

Executives still get ulcers – the fashionable adjective applied to them now is not duodenal or gastric but 'peptic' – but they don't boast about them the way they used to, maybe because a remarkable pharmaceutical discovery in the 1970s made their treatment much simpler and far less dramatic.

Something that puzzled me when I first learned biology, and was taught that our stomachs and intestines produced powerful enzymes and acid that could digest the toughest of meat, was why we didn't digest our own insides. The reason, I discovered, is that the whole of our digestive tract is lined with a protective membrane – the slippery mucous membrane you can feel when you run your tongue around the inside of your cheek.

If that membrane is breached, as can happen when you catch your cheek on a sharp tooth or inadvertently bite it, the digestive enzymes in your saliva attack the underlying tissue until the mucous lining grows slowly back to protect it. And, during that time, you will have a painful ulcer in your mouth.

A duodenal ulcer develops in much the same way. The duodenum is the first portion of the small intestine that food enters after it leaves the stomach, and there our food is digested not just by powerful enzymes produced by the pancreas but by other enzymes and acid that the food brings with it from the stomach. When a breach occurs in the mucous membrane lining the duodenum, an ulcer occurs in much the same way that it does in our mouths, save that the digestive juices that act on the underlying tissue are much more powerful than those in our saliva and are abetted by the acid that has come from the stomach.

The common cause of a breach in the duodenum's protective lining is an excess flow of irritant acid from the stomach. Excess acid may be provoked by rushed irregular meals which leave little time for the peaceful digestion of food and are common ingredients of a busy executive existence. Add other excess acid provokers, like drinking on an empty stomach and smoking, and you have the perfect recipe for producing an ulcer.

As a duodenal ulcer develops, it can cause severe pain and discomfort and, if the digestive juices erode the wall of a blood vessel, they may cause bleeding. If they erode their way right through the wall of the duodenum, the ulcer perforates and germs which normally reside quite harmlessly within the intestine escape into the abdominal cavity to cause infection – peritonitis.

The treatment of duodenal ulcers has always been designed not just to stop the pain but to encourage the ulcer to heal quickly and prevent it progressing to the point where it may cause bleeding or will perforate. The main barrier to healing is the acid which flows into the duodenum from the stomach and fifteen years ago nearly all treatments involved a regular intake of powders and milk to neutralise the acid, and sufferers had to stick to bland diets which were not only anti-acid but free from irritants like spices which might aggravate the ulcer.

To prevent a build-up of acid, doctors advised patients to eat 'a little and often' and to seek 'peace of mind' – a state more easily described than achieved. Sufferers were also told to avoid 'noxious influences' – smoking, alcohol and coffee – which were thought to delay an ulcer's healing.

Patients with persistent ulcers were admitted to hospital where rest in bed, isolation from the stress of the outside world, and, sometimes sedation, accelerated the healing of their ulcers. Some with recurrent ulcers had part of their stomachs removed –

the part that produces the acid. Others had an operation to block the nerves involved in acid production.

The first drug treatments were concerned exclusively with neutralising the acid. Later came drugs designed to reduce the production of acid but, though these worked, they were not as effective as doctors would have liked.

The first drug shown scientifically to accelerate ulcer healing was a derivative of liquorice, carbenoxelone, which appeared in the early 1970s. Yet although it healed the ulcers more quickly, the patient's pain and discomfort were slow to go, probably because these were still being caused by the high acid levels which caused the ulcer in the first place.

The real breakthrough in treatment came with the discovery of drugs called H_2-receptor antagonists. Their complicated name is a scientific description of the way they work but what is important from the sufferer's point of view is the result. Given in the right dose, these easily swallowed tablets inhibit the production of stomach acid very effectively and for long periods. And they've been found not just to accelerate the healing of the ulcer but to relieve the sufferer's discomfort rapidly, usually within a few days of starting treatment.

The most commonly used drugs in this group are cimetidine and ranitidine and friends of mine who once suffered badly from ulcers tell me the effect of the drugs is 'magical'. They have said goodbye to recurrent episodes of pain and one or two whose ulcers have flared up after treatment have been able to return to work, firing on all cylinders, much earlier than they'd ever done before.

Other patients have even managed to avoid recurrences since their doctors put them on a maintenance dosage. But no one should do that for themselves. Indeed these drugs should always be taken under medical supervision. The supervising doctor needs to do tests to ensure that the indigestion is being caused by an ulcer and not by something else, and also needs to monitor treatment to ensure that patients are not subjected to any unnecessary risk of haemorrhage or perforation.

Cimetidine and ranitidine have revolutionised ulcer treatment but some sufferers are still burdened with advice about their lifestyle which is a hangover from times past. A lot of this advice about the virtues of a 'bland diet' and the dangers of alcohol and 'stress' is backed by little evidence. The only villain fingered by the evidence is smoking which has been shown not only to impair the healing of an ulcer but to encourage its recurrence and thus increase the likelihood that it will have to be treated with surgery.

As for diet, it's clearly sensible for ulcer sufferers to avoid foods which they know precipitate their symptoms but there is no scientific justification for a total ban on alcohol – though some may find it helps to switch from spirits to wine or beer. There's also no scientific evidence that ulcers are linked to stress: it's the smoking and irregular eating that go with the stress that cause the trouble.

The new drugs have greatly reduced the number of patients needing operations for their ulcers; just as our increased knowledge of the non-links between ulcers and lifestyle have reduced the vocabulary of executive boasting. Yet most executives, I'm sure, will be happy to forgo the status symbol as long as they can also forgo the pain, the discomfort, and the risks.

| Positive action |

Recurrent dyspepsia is not an essential ingredient of business life. If you suffer from it, seek medical advice. Remember that though we now have effective treatments for ulcers, they still occur.

You can't reap the benefits of modern treatment – for dyspepsia as well as ulcers – if you don't consult a doctor. The constant chewing of 'indigestion tablets' was OK behaviour for a tycoon in an ancient Hollywood movie; in the 1980s, it smacks of foolishness.

Hangovers: an occupational hazard of selling

Swedes refer to it as *Hont i haret* – pain in the hair roots; in Norway they say *Jeg har tommermen* – I have carpenters in the head. Germans call it *Katzenjammer* – the wailing of cats, and in

Britain we call it a hangover. A London psychiatrist once objected to my writing about its treatment in a newspaper because he thought that, by offering alleviation to the afflicted, I was encouraging over-indulgence in the cause.

I understand his concern (and so may you when you read *The trouble with booze* on page 139). That psychiatrist spends much of his time trying to salvage lives which have been wrecked by addiction to alcohol. Yet I feel justified in writing about hangovers on this page because for many a businessman and woman they are not a symptom of addiction but an occupational injury. I remember a business executive who was a patient of mine complaining that he got his worst hangovers when he hadn't enjoyed the company he'd been forced to keep the night before. 'It's unfair,' he said, 'to be punished when you haven't even enjoyed yourself.'

To appease the psychiatrist, and my own conscience, before I deal with the occupational injury – the hangover – I must consider the occupational disease – alcohol addiction: particularly because business executives are one of the groups known to be at highest risk. The levels of consumption which indicate you could be damaging your health are spelled out on page 143. If you regularly exceed those levels, hangovers are the least of your problems and, instead of reading on, you should lay this book aside, pick up a telephone, and make an appointment with your doctor.

For those of you whose regular drinking is below the danger limits, a hangover is probably an occasional injury suffered at a sales conference or an international congress. Or it could be an affliction which strikes after a night out with the boys, or after one of those business meetings at which a deal could be reached only by following the client into the world of his own indulgence.

Businessmen's hangovers are compounded of several ingredients. Alcohol is a powerful sedative drug and appears to be a stimulant only because the first layer of the brain it sedates is that which exercises civilised control over the less sophisticated layers. Its initial effect is to disinhibit behaviour but, as its concentration in the brain rises, so it produces sleepiness and eventually a 'knock-out' coma.

Like other sedatives, alcohol drugs the brain cells and when it is withdrawn, the cells take time to recover. That recovery is one element of a hangover. Another is the toxic effect produced on brain cells by aromatic substances called congeners which give drinks their individual flavours.

Yet another element is dehydration. Alcohol stimulates the kidneys and if, for instance, you drink a pint of beer, it stimulates you to pass more than a pint of urine. That is why bar room doors have such well worn hinges and why an evening's drinking can tilt the water balance of our bodies into debt, producing a dry mouth and a particularly nasty form of headache.

If you have been drinking heavily on an empty stomach, a gastric upset may also be part of your hangover and another common element is lack of proper sleep. You probably were late to bed and much of your sleep may have been that dreamless alcoholic near-coma which does little to refresh the brain.

Positive action

What can we do to prevent the harmful elements in alcohol from building up?

- a worthwhile gambit is to try to slow down alcohol absorption by drinking a glass of milk before you start: enthusiasts use olive oil. This ploy may also protect you against gastric upset by preventing the alcohol from irritating your stomach lining.

- unless you've been drinking very heavily, you'll find that the nastiest ingredient of your hangover is dehydration. You can often prevent this if you drink at least half a litre of water before you go to bed – and also take a couple of soluble aspirin. A less dramatic way is to have a bottle of water on the dinner table alongside the wine to remind you to keep drinking it.

- you can try to stop the build up of congeners by not mixing your drinks and avoiding – or going easy on – drinks which are high on congeners: red wine, brandy, and port. Drinks low on congeners include white wine, white rum, and vodka (less likely to give you a headache than gin). If you choose your drinks unwisely, you can ease the 'morning after' headache by taking honey which speeds the elimination of congeners.

If you've been drinking really heavily, preventive action won't work completely. You may prevent the dehydration but, as the alcohol level in your brain begins to subside, you may experience bouts of nausea and that odd disorientation, often described as a feeling of walking six inches above the ground, that comes as your brain cells try to re-establish their normal activities.

This state can be partially alleviated – though not cured – by decelerating the rate at which the alcohol level is falling. Hence the traditional cure of 'a hair of the dog' – another drink – though that carries the danger of encouraging further drinking which will set you up for another, even worse, hangover.

Most traditional hangover cures – Prairie Oyster, Fernet Branca, your favourite barman's special remedy – use small doses of alcohol to slow the 'sobering up' of your brain cells and give them more time to recover. Many of the 'cures' seem also to include a masochistic element, tasting so nasty that you feel you are making suitable penance for the sinning of the night before.

I have to admit, however, that neither bartenders nor doctors have yet found the answer to the king-size hangover that yields only to the passage of time and for which the American humorist Robert Benchley once suggested that the only cure was death.

A useful tip

The only sure way of preventing a hangover is not to drink at all. Yet refusing a drink seems often to challenge a client or customer into forcing you to have one. And persistent refusal may threaten a useful relationship you've spent a lot of time and effort establishing.

It's now common knowledge that people who've suffered a liver complaint are forbidden to drink for a long time afterwards. Also, maybe because it is seen as an Act of God rather than a self-inflicted injury, a 'liver complaint' is an OK complaint for an executive to admit to – and more likely to evoke sympathy than doubts about physical fitness.

So an acceptable excuse for sticking to soft drinks all evening or through lunch – and, in some circles, it is the only acceptable excuse – is to refer with a sigh to 'this liver trouble' and to explain that your doctor won't let you touch the stuff.

You'll find that that deceit – acceptable surely because it harms nobody – will deter even the most persistent from forcing drinks on you.

Middle-aged eyes

When a friend of mine was elevated to the board of a London bank, his ten-year-old nephew was delighted. 'Now when you go on television,' he said, 'they'll give you a pair of those cut-in-half glasses.'

It's not surprising a child should think that half spectacles are a symbol of status. The long-sightedness that makes them necessary usually asserts itself at an age when men and women acquire more substantial symbols of achievement in their work. Indeed one ophthalmic surgeon I know says the age at which we all become long-sighted is remarkably constant. If a mature person comes to him seeking glasses, he asks if their last birthday was their forty-eighth. The commonest answer he gets is: 'How did you know?'

If you have reached that magic age, you may well have noticed that you need to hold books or papers further from you than you once did and that even a restaurant menu has to be held at arm's length to be decipherable. This long-sightedness develops because the shape of our eyes alters as we grow older and the muscles that control the lens can no longer focus it on nearby objects. The usual remedy is 'reading glasses' which can be worn only for close work and which, when not in use, are easily – and usually – mislaid.

Three fashionable solutions to the problems of mislaying your spectacles are to suspend them from a cord or chain around the neck (though I have a friend who still indulges in the traditional hunt for her glasses having forgotten they dangle on her bosom), pushing the spectacles up on to the forehead (a manoeuvre much

An insight that came almost too late

William Jones, aged fifty-six, though far from a soap opera character, always dictated his letters in the style of a soap opera tycoon. He strode up and down his office, pausing only when in search of a word.

One day, when in full flow, he tripped over a small space heater and gashed his forehead on a corner of his desk. A doctor was summoned and, after he had dressed the wound, he asked William if he'd had any trouble with his eyesight.

Funny he should ask, said William.

He'd always had good eyesight. Before he'd damaged his shoulder he'd been a first class tennis player with a 'good eye' for the ball.

But recently he'd been having a little trouble. Nothing serious, just a feeling that at times his vision was not quite as good as it ought to be, especially when the light was poor. He was thinking of having his eyes tested to see if he needed spectacles.

The doctor gave him the name of a local ophthalmologist who, when he tested William, found he had lost virtually all his peripheral vision. The damage to his sight was irreversible and, without treatment, would have progressed until he became blind.

William also learned that, if he had had a routine check-up of his eyes when he was fifty, he need not have lost the amount of vision that he had. The need for prevention so impressed him that every executive in his company now receives a special birthday card on his fiftieth birthday. William offers them his best wishes and recommends that they go and have their eyes tested.

Most of them appreciate that he's not trying to insult them.

favoured by news editors in movies) and the half spectacles that allow the wearer to peer over them at distant objects and use the lenses to look at nearby ones.

Half spectacles are often favoured by men who reach the upper echelons of business because, when used skilfully, they endow the wearer with the appurtenances – if not the actuality – of shrewdness, or even wisdom.

The coming of long-sightedness poses particular problems for those who are already short-sighted and who may have been wearing spectacles for most of their lives. It is one of Sod's Laws of Nature that the two conditions do not cancel one another out and when short-sighted people reach middle age they often acquire two pairs of spectacles to mislay.

Another affliction of middle-aged eyes, more serious than the rather jokey long-sightedness, is glaucoma. The disease occurs in several forms and the commonest afflicts about 2 per cent of people in Britain aged over forty. It is an insidiously progressive disease which, if untreated, will lead to eventual blindness. Yet, if it is detected early, simple treatment with eye drops can prevent the loss of vision.

The nasty thing about this common form of glaucoma is that, in its early stages, it produces no symptoms and gives no sign of its existence. Yet, by the time it is detected, the damage it has done cannot be repaired. That is why ophthalmologists recommend that everyone have their eyes tested at the age of fifty – younger if they are at special risk.

The central disorder in glaucoma is a rise of pressure within the eye. Normally, the fluid that fills the eyeball is constantly, though slowly, replaced, and the excess drains away through a filter-bed which lies around the edge of the iris – the coloured diaphragm that surrounds the pupil.

In people with the common sort of glaucoma, the filter-bed gets clogged by progressive microscopic changes, and the slowing down of drainage causes a rise of fluid pressure within the eye. The raised pressure compresses the tiny blood vessels that carry oxygen to the optic nerve – the nerve which carries visual images to the brain – and tiny filaments of the nerve then die.

The first bits of nerve to go lie close to the 'blind spot' – the tiny natural gap we all have in our vision. Our eyes are conditioned to ignore this gap so when people with glaucoma first start to lose vision, their eyes treat the loss as if it were an extension of the blind spot and the victim remains completely unaware of what is happening.

Only later, when the peripheral vision starts to go, will people get a vague feeling that their eyesight is not as good as it was, or they start to bump into things they once would have seen or to trip over minor obstacles in their path. By then it is too late to prevent a serious loss of nerve tissue, and of vision.

Some people run an increased risk of the disease. The biggest risk is inheritance. Recent studies suggest it will occur in about 10 per cent of the close relatives of an affected person and ophthalmologists now try to examine the eyes of members of the family of every patient.

People also run an increased risk if they have diabetes or raised blood pressure. Ophthalmologists recommend that they, like the close relatives of glaucoma patients, should have their eyes tested regularly from around the age of forty-five or even forty. Modern tests can now detect the disease at a much earlier stage than was possible only ten years ago.

When glaucoma is detected early, its progress can be halted with eyedrops that reduce the pressure within the eyeball. (With the most up-to-date drops some patients can get round-the-clock control of pressure using just one drop twice a day.) Other patients may need an operation performed with a laser.

The most important message about glaucoma, however, is not that ophthalmologists can now treat it effectively but that, if they see it early, they can prevent its damaging effects.

Positive action

The onset of long-sightedness in middle age is a useful reminder of the need to have a test for glaucoma.

- if a close relative has suffered from glaucoma, you should have your eyes tested regularly from your early forties

- if you are a diabetic, you should have your eyes tested from your early forties

- anyone who's never had an eye test should have one before their fiftieth birthday

The danger of being 'hard of hearing'

Success in business can bring one penalty that rarely gets publicity. The higher a person rises in the hierarchy of a company, the less easily can he or she admit to any form of physical weakness.

At each level of promotion the competition grows tougher and people are disinclined to own up to a disability which, though it has no effect on their efficiency, might just count against them when their worth is assessed against others of near-equal talent and achievement.

Sometimes the attempts at concealment continue long after the disability is obvious to all and the result can be bizarre.

I once sat on a committee chaired by a man who was seriously deaf yet was not prepared to admit it. Every member of that committee knew the chairman was deaf because we all had to speak loudly if we wanted him to hear – and softly if we didn't – yet he maintained the charade that he could hear everything perfectly.

His life, and ours, would have been much easier if he had been prepared to wear a hearing aid but that would have subverted the macho image that he liked to project. A hearing aid would have proclaimed: 'I have a physical defect', and his reluctance to wear one was not just a matter of personal vanity but a reflection of the attitude most of us have towards deafness.

Few comedians or cartoonists would make a joke that mocked the disability of someone who was blind. Yet the deaf are regular butts of such jokes even though any doctor or nurse who has worked with both deaf and blind people will tell you that deafness is the worse disability.

One reason for our attitude is that we can communicate with the blind. We can express our sympathy and try to help them without putting too great a strain upon ourselves. We don't have to expend too much effort in order to get that warm glow of satisfaction that comes from 'doing good'.

In people who are deaf, however, their disability gets between them and us.

Unless they have learned to lip read, we grow frustrated as we try to communicate with them. Our reward is not a warm glow of satisfaction but irritation. And the repetitive shouting in which we have to engage to get them to understand leads us to behave as if we are dealing with people who are not deaf but stupid.

That image of the 'difficult' deaf person can haunt successful business executives who become 'hard of hearing' in their late fifties or early sixties. And, because they don't wish to acknowledge their disability, they deny themselves access to medical help that could make their lives much easier.

Let's analyse their position in the way they would analyse a business problem. First marshal the data and then sketch out possible solutions.

The data

We all suffer a loss of hearing as we grow older, though some lose more than others. Most just suffer a slight loss of the subtlety of hearing; a few, particularly if they had an infection of their ears when they were young, find it difficult to hear normal conversation.

The reason for this loss of hearing is a loss of efficiency in the nerves which carry impulses from the ear, where they are generated, to the brain, which interprets them as sound.

But this loss of efficiency caused by natural ageing is not the only cause of deafness. By far the commonest cause is obstruction of the outer ear by a lump of the wax which our ears produce to trap dust that might otherwise travel downwards and irritate the drum. Less commonly, deafness can be caused by infections, which can be treated with antibiotics or sometimes by surgery, or by rare diseases of the middle ear whose effects can be countered by delicate surgery.

Positive action

First seek medical advice. Don't go straight to a hearing aid salesman.

The likeliest cause of your loss of hearing is a lump of wax in your outer ear. Wax is easily removed and only when it's gone

Wear your badge proudly

One of the most moving radio talks I've heard was given by Richard Leech, an actor of great talent who has had, and is still having, a distinguished career in the theatre and in films and television.

Before he became an actor, he trained as a doctor so when, as a young man, he started to go deaf, he knew whom to consult and which tests he needed. He discovered that he had a rare form of deafness which was inevitably progressive and for which nothing could be done.

He accepted his condition with extraordinary stoicism and continued his career. He learned to lip read on stage and, as his hearing deteriorated, devised ways of coping with particular problems.

If he couldn't hear one of his cues from off-stage, he would get a stage hand to tap him on the shoulder when the words were spoken and then stride on briskly, often to answer a question he had never heard being asked.

He decided early on that he would never wear a hearing aid. Wearing one, he said, was a form of capitulation. One day a doctor friend told him he was being foolishly pig-headed. So he decided to try an aid and the broadcast talk I heard was an exhortation to others not to be as stupid as he had been.

His hearing aid, he said, had transformed his life, returned him from isolation to the world of others, and allowed him to drop ridiculous tricks in which he'd indulged in a feeble attempt to conceal his disability. He'd decided to wear his aid not with shame but with pride in the hope it might encourage others.

Richard Leech's message applies not only to those who, like himself, have a serious hearing disability but to those who admit, if only to themselves, to being hard of hearing.

will you realise how long it's been there. Anyone who has had wax syringed from their ears will tell you of their magical re-entry to the world when they suddenly re-heard sounds they had forgotten existed.

If your loss of hearing is the sort of deterioration that afflicts us as we grow older, it can be countered by using a hearing aid to amplify the sounds entering the ear.

Don't shy away from the thought of a hearing aid. Minia-turised electronics have allowed a great variety of design. Modern aids can be hidden in spectacle frames or tucked discreetly into the outer ear.

For anyone whose hearing has grown gradually blunted, a hearing aid can bring that magical re-entry to the world that others experience when their ears are cleared of wax.

The way to find the hearing aid best adapted to your needs is to first consult an ear specialist and seek his or her advice. Not only will you get independent advice on the cosmetic possibilities but you will also be advised on the range of sounds that you need amplified.

I find it sad that so many people whose lives could be made much easier and more enjoyable by a hearing aid are not prepared to use one because they've never had the courage – and I admit it does take courage – to find out what's available.

Investigating the possibilities doesn't commit you to using a hearing aid but just experiencing the benefit could persuade you.

Depression is a dirty word

We all feel depressed at times without there being any question of us suffering from a mental illness, and we usually shake off the mood by 'pulling ourselves together'.

There is, however, a form of depression which is an illness, and one that afflicts one in twenty-five people at some time in their lives. Indeed recent investigations suggest that in Britain it affects one in twenty people visiting a GP's surgery.

And it can kill.

Yet the symptoms of this potentially fatal disease often go

undetected by those around the sufferer. When it causes suicide, people who knew the victim well may think retrospectively that maybe for a few weeks he – or she – had tended to take a gloomy view of things and, on occasion, had been uncharacteristically morose. But not to any extent that would worry them. For much of the time those who are most dangerously ill can appear to be their usual cheerful selves.

And that's why pathological depression is such a dangerous disease, particularly in people who are their own bosses, or who work in positions where they have no one in the company hierarchy in whom they can confide without losing face or harming their chances of promotion. People who live highly competitive lives become clever at concealing their true emotions even from their closest companions.

The pathological depression that kills is not the simple emotion that we all feel. Nor is it a reaction to depressing events – though it may seem to be. It is caused by some change *within* the person who suffers it, probably a minute change in the biochemical processes in the brain.

And while most of us can shrug off an attack of the 'blues', pathological depression won't go away. Indeed a good definition of its central feature is the loss of the capacity to 'pull yourself together'.

When the illness is not too severe people who regularly suffer from it can recognise its arrival. Winston Churchill used to announce that the 'black dog' had taken up residence. Like other victims, he then kept himself going by constantly reminding himself that, no matter how deep the depression was, it always went away. The black dog never fails to leave the house, though its departure is often just as mysterious and unpredictable as its arrival.

Yet when the depression is severe, the victims lose insight into what is happening to them. Their outlook on the world becomes wholly gloomy and they suffer profound feelings of guilt. They grow certain they will never get better and, as they sink into despair, they are at very real risk. Depressive illness is the cause of two thirds of all suicides.

The risk is especially high in people who are suffering from the

Everything to live for

William Marsh was a successful entrepreneur.

When he left school he got a job as a typewriter salesman and later started a small office supplies business which grew into a retail chain with some eighty outlets.

By the age of forty-one, he was not just a successful businessman but happily married and had two teenage children to whom he was a kind and indulgent father. He claimed with pride that he ran his small headquarters office as a 'family business'. Most of his staff had been with him for a long time, he treated them well, and they were intensely loyal.

Then one evening, after what had seemed to everyone around him to be a normal working day, he walked down to the local railway line and threw himself under a train.

The inquest heard that he was under no special stress at home or at work and that his business affairs were in good order. His suicide came as a shock to everyone who knew him. 'Unbelievable,' they said. 'He had reaped the benefits of years of hard work and had everything to live for.'

The coroner's verdict was that he had killed himself 'while the balance of his mind was disturbed'.

William's story is not an uncommon one. You may have seen the short paragraphs in local newspapers. People with apparently rewarding lives ahead of them suddenly, and for no obvious reason, destroy themselves. The paragraphs are headstones beneath which are buried stories every bit as tragic as that of William Marsh.

And in most of the stories, as in William's, the traditional formula of the coroner's verdict is literally true. The balance of their minds is disturbed by a depressive illness . . .

illness for the first time and who give little indication to the outside world of the torment raging within. They do not recognise that they are ill because to them their depression is an exaggeration of a mood we are all used to accepting as part of a normal life.

If you could put an evil 'fluence on the next three people you pass in the street and make them depressed, all would have some good reason for being so. People who suffer from pathological depression don't see their reaction as abnormal but fix their attention wholly on one of those reasons we all have for feeling depressed.

That is why many of them never seek help and why, if they do screw up their courage and confide in others, the listeners may accept the reasons they offer for being depressed and fail to recognise the severity of the illness which lies beneath.

Only later do relatives and friends realise how out of proportion the depression was to its apparent cause, how obsessed the sufferer seemed with a worry which he or she would normally have shrugged off. Sadly, that realisation by relatives and friends is nearly always retrospective and often comes too late.

The tragedy of depressive illness is that the deaths it causes are unnecessary. The depression always clears itself eventually yet the victim may kill himself – or herself – before it has time to do so.

The tragedy seems even greater now that doctors can use anti-depressant drugs to alleviate the illness until it resolves. These drugs are not tranquillisers but drugs that seem to act specifically on the biochemical processes that underlie the depression.

The existence of effective treatment makes it vital that people suffering from pathological depression be given the chance to see a doctor for assessment.

You should suspect its presence in others if their depth of depression seems out of proportion to its apparent cause, if they seem to harbour exaggerated feelings of guilt, or if their normal depressive reaction to some tragedy, like a bereavement, continues for much longer than you would normally expect.

You may recognise it in yourself if you find you have a depression you can't shake off, if it is at its worst when you first wake in the morning and lightens as the day progresses, if it disturbs your sleep pattern so you tend to wake in the early hours, if it is associated with loss of energy and with loss of appetite for food and sex.

With depression, it is often difficult to draw the line between the normal and abnormal. If in doubt, seek medical advice. Sadly, many executives are not prepared to accept that their depression is a disease. And, for some, that decision is fatal.

Nagging Afflictions

Good night

The journal *World Medicine* once ran a survey to discover what were the commonest questions that people ask of off-duty doctors. The winner, by a mile, was: 'Now look here, doc. What can I do to be sure of a good night's sleep?'

Executives under pressure, working irregular hours and maybe travelling through time zones, are almost guaranteed to have disrupted sleep patterns and their chief worry about insomnia is that it may blunt their competitive edge the following day. Some take sleeping tablets; some learn to live with disrupted sleep. Only a few consider it a serious enough problem for a formal visit to a doctor; many more think it just the sort of subject to raise conversationally in a locker room or bar.

Sleep is an odd condition and, although most of us spend about a third of our lives indulging in it, scientists have until recently known very little about what happens to our bodies while we're asleep.

All living creatures have a pattern of activity and inactivity related to the appearance and disappearance of the sun which in regular 24-hour cycles varies our environment between light combined with warmth and darkness combined with cold.

This cyclical pattern produces a response from every tissue in our bodies. Throughout our lives these tissues are in a state of constant change as they wear out and are replaced. Over each 24-hour cycle, wearing out and replacement balance each other but wearing out dominates while we are awake and replacement dominates while we are asleep.

Chemical changes in the body reflect this pattern. Measurements of hormones, for instance, show that the ones that are dominant during wakefulness are those, such as adrenalin and cortisol, which are associated not just with tissue breakdown but also with achievement. During sleep these hormones are at a low level and dominated by the growth hormone and other tissue-building hormones.

These cyclical body changes can affect businessmen who are forced to work irregular hours, or to fly across time zones, and who thus face the same problems as shift workers – a group which has recently been the subject of much scientific study.

On their days off, shift workers like to be up and about at the same time as everybody else, so they never adapt fully to either a working or rest day pattern. If they try to sleep during the day, their body temperature rises at the usual clock time instead of falling as it should do during sleep, and their hormone balance is often at cross-purposes with their physical activities. If they never get time to adapt to a single pattern, they may suffer from digestive and stress disorders.

The same problems may afflict executives who radically change their work patterns or who travel east or west by air. To adapt to the new sleep/wakefulness pattern, their bodies will need roughly one day for every hour of time difference. (See page 49, *Coping with jet lag*.)

Less dramatic than 'jet lag' but no less irksome are other sleep problems which afflict businessmen and women. The commonest is a form of insomnia which affects people working under pressure and is usually expressed as: 'I don't seem to be able to get as much sleep as I'd like and it's beginning to wear me out.'

The anxiety generated by this sort of insomnia is based on a misunderstanding. Our bodies will always take as much sleep as they need and the fatigue that many people feel after a 'bad night' comes not from lack of sleep but because their energy has been drained during the night by the anxiety that afflicted them during the lonely spells of wakefulness.

Ironically, that anxiety is often over how awful they're going to feel the following day and how difficult they're going to find it to cope with one of tomorrow's problems because they can't get to sleep now.

Just by reminding themselves that exhaustive scientific research has shown that a 'sleepless night' – no nights are completely sleepless even though many feel they are – will not take away their competitive edge next day, they might relieve their anxiety and slip into a relaxing slumber.

Research in university sleep laboratories – where people are observed and their bodies' electrical and chemical activities monitored while they are asleep – has not only shown that insomniacs spend much less time awake than they think but has given rise to the quaint phrase 'sleep hygiene' to describe behaviour that helps people to enjoy their sleep.

Positive action

Sleep researchers' tips to improve sleep hygiene include:

- do something absorbing and relaxing in the hour before you go to bed. Special relaxation exercises can help.

- train yourself to a sleep rhythm by setting an alarm to wake you at the same time every day and by not indulging in 'sleep-ins' on days off.

- stay up until you feel sleepy, even if this means staying up very late. If you find you're not getting off to sleep, get up and do something absorbing, like reading, in another room until you feel sleepy. In this way you will avoid associating your bedroom, and your bed, with sleeplessness.

- above all remind yourself there is no evidence that everyone needs eight hours' sleep a night. Your body will take all the sleep it needs. Sleep hygiene is designed only to make the hours you spend in bed more comfortable.

If you follow these simple tips, you may at first get occasional spells of sleepiness during the day but these will soon pass and, as you establish a rhythm, your bad nights will gradually be replaced by good ones.

Coping with pain

Most of us suffer occasional pains – usually headaches or back-aches – which, while we have them, can make us less efficient at our work, less tolerant, more irritable.

Yet business executives – possibly because of the competitive world in which they live – tend to regard the idea of taking a pain reliever as some sort of weakness, as though the business-like thing is to 'soldier on' until the pain disappears, despite its effect on their efficiency and concentration.

I think they are misguided.

There's enough 'suffering' involved in trying to succeed in business without having to endure the distraction of unnecessary pain, particularly these days when a wide range of pain relievers is available for all degrees of pain.

Modern medical science can supply you with effective pain relief whether your pain be severe or niggling, acute or chronic.

For severe pain the treatment will be prescribed by a doctor because the stronger pain relievers are available only on pre-scription. One reason for controlling their supply is the need for the cause of severe pain to be established. If the cause is serious, it may need treatment just as urgently because the pain, though disabling, is only a symptom or signal that something is wrong. You don't, however, need to consult a doctor about every pain. The commonest forms of pain from which most of us suffer could be called 'household pains': occasional headaches, backaches, muscular strains and twinges, the irritating rawness of nose and throat we get with a cold.

Yet though they're not serious, household pains can reduce our efficiency if we just 'soldier on' with them. Better by far to make ourselves more comfortable by taking a humble remedy which has been around so long – since 1899 – that we've come to take it for granted.

The original household remedy

Even in the age of 'wonder drugs', aspirin is still an effective remedy for everyday aches and pains. It's particularly useful

An example of true courage

One of the most heroic men I ever met led what must have seemed to many the least heroic of lives.

He was financial director of a small engineering company and, for the nineteen years that I knew him, worked the same regular hours in the same office block in the same corner of suburban London. He was kind to his staff, rarely lost his temper, and the nearest he came to boasting was when he told me that, while he knew his work was unimaginative, he hoped it was competent.

Only his wife, a few close friends, and I, his doctor, knew that he suffered continual pain – not severe but unremitting.

I awarded him the accolade of heroism because he managed to preserve not just his efficiency but his personal equanimity while suffering pain which I knew interfered with his sleep and concentration and from which he knew there was little prospect of relief.

That was twenty-five years ago.

Today, thanks to dramatic though largely unsung advances in medical knowledge, no one needs to emulate his heroism.

because it's not just a pain-killer. It can also make us more comfortable during diseases like influenza by lowering our fever, and is still one of the most effective reducers of inflammation in the joints of people with arthritis.

Yet though doctors, and their patients, have known for nearly ninety years just how useful it is, only recently have scientists been able to produce a convincing theory to explain *how* it works – and many would say they need to discover much more before we can completely understand it.

All we know for certain is that it affects a group of hormone-like substances called prostaglandins which are found in many tissues of the body and which play a part in the control of pain, and possibly in regulating body temperature.

Another unusual quality of aspirin is that, despite its use by billions of people since the beginning of this century, it has proved to be remarkably free from side-effects. The announcement a few years ago that, when given to young children, it might cause an extremely rare neurological condition called Reye's syndrome seemed so much at odds with aspirin's normal character that it became front-page news.

That risk is unlikely to deter those who rely on aspirin as an easer of mundane discomforts. For them its only drawback is its irritant effect on the lining of the stomach. This irritation can cause 'heartburn' and indigestion, and in rare cases – about one in every 6,500 'heavy users' – may cause bleeding. Most people try to counter this irritant effect by taking it with food or by using a soluble form.

The greatest danger with aspirin is that, because it is the most widely used pain-killer in the world and because it can be found in nearly every household, we don't always treat it with the respect it deserves.

The observance of a few dogmatic rules would eliminate most of the few risks associated with this most useful of drugs:

- never take aspirin on an empty stomach or if you suffer from a gastric or a duodenal ulcer. I find the best way to avoid its dyspeptic effects is to take it in soluble form

- if you suffer from diabetes or are on anti-coagulant drugs, never take aspirin without first consulting a doctor

- if you have to take aspirin for more than a couple of days, consult your doctor: the condition you are trying to relieve may need medical investigation

- don't give aspirin to children without first getting a doctor's advice

- don't exceed the maximum dosage recommended on the package

- keep your supply out of the reach of children. Aspirin can be dangerous in gross overdosage

If you take those simple precautions, you can rely on aspirin to relieve those irksome symptoms which can impair working efficiency without being serious enough to need professional attention: headaches, limb aches, or joint aches caused, among other things, by fatigue, a head cold, excess humidity, sitting cramped in a crowded plane or train, or the after-effects of an unaccustomed dose of exercise or alcohol.

The next time you're plagued by one of those everyday afflictions of business life, you can reach for the bottle of aspirin, confident that you are reaching for a remedy that has been on test since Victoria was queen.

Other household remedies

Aspirin is a popular remedy because people have found it works and it is an ingredient of nearly every pain-killer that finds its way into bathroom cupboards. These days those cupboards may contain two other drugs which have proved useful for relieving everyday aches and pains, particularly in people who are allergic to aspirin.

The first is ibuprofen, available from chemists under the trade name Nurofen. It acts in much the same way as aspirin and is useful for relieving pain caused by inflamed joints and muscles.

The second is paracetamol, which has now been around for thirty years and which, unlike aspirin, doesn't cause gastric irritation. But it doesn't have aspirin's anti-inflammatory effect and is therefore less effective in relieving arthritic pain and other pains associated with inflammation.

Paracetamol can cause serious liver damage when taken in overdose. This damage is often irreversible and can be fatal, so the tablets should be kept well out of the reach of children.

Other pain-killers available without prescription usually have aspirin or paracetamol as their main ingredient. Those with an image of 'greater power' have it endowed by their advertising rather than by their ingredients.

This doesn't mean you shouldn't try them. Response to pain-killers is highly individual and if you find one that suits you, then stick with it. Those that are on sale without prescription have few side-effects – otherwise their sale would be restricted – and all carry warnings about these on the packet.

Coping with more serious pain

Never put up with pain which hangs around for more than three days or continues unremittingly for 24 hours despite treatment with household remedies. That sort of pain needs medical investigation.

Just as important, never let the fear of pain prevent you from having a medical investigation.

The good news to emerge from the technological progress made over the past decade and a half is that today no one should have to put up with severe pain. Modern medical and dental treatment should be pain free. If you find it isn't, you should ask why – and don't accept an excuse as an answer.

Even incurable disease should no longer produce severe pain. Modern techniques and a vastly improved knowledge of methods of pain control allow doctors to relieve every form of pain that man is heir to.

Ironically, most of the severe pain suffered today is self-inflicted because people brought up in the 'soldiering on' tradition refuse to accept the help that is available because they fear being 'drugged'.

The 'soldiering on' attitude is common among those who've succeeded in highly competitive business. Executives who have won success by overcoming challenges see illness and pain as yet another challenge which they want to deal with on their own without any outside help.

I understand the attitude but find it sad because the technological advances in pain control have been so great that many NHS hospitals now have specialist clinics devoted not to treating particular illnesses but to treating pain, whatever its cause.

Our growing knowledge of the biochemical mechanisms which underlie pain has led to the development of new drugs, of refined forms of acupuncture, of ways of electronically stimulating nerves to produce our own natural pain-killing endorphins, and of surgical techniques designed to block the nerves that carry pain-producing impulses.

These days no one need suffer severe pain and the days of heroic suffering are over. They have been banished not just by

Two major steps towards understanding pain

Over the past fifteen years, medical scientists have greatly expanded our knowledge of the biochemical mechanisms through which pain is produced.

In particular, they have unravelled two processes which provide opportunities for preventing and relieving pain.

Billions of microscopic pain receptors exist in the skin and in most organs. They are front-line defences, sensitive to any potentially harmful stimulation. When triggered by injury or irritation, they send warning signals along nerves to our brains where the signals are interpreted as pain.

Recently scientists have discovered that, when the receptors are stimulated, cells around them release chemicals – the best known are called prostaglandins – into the bloodstream. And when these chemicals reach the brain, they lower the body's pain threshold – the level at which a sensation becomes painful.

Scientists now suspect that certain kinds of pain, such as those produced by arthritis and migraine, are linked with this chemical lowering of sensitivity.

The second discovery is that powerful pain relievers like morphine work by attaching themselves to special sites on the surface of brain cells. Clearly those sites don't exist for the convenience of outside drugs like morphine and their discoverers assumed they were intended for naturally-occurring brain chemicals with which the body could protect itself against pain. They have since identified those chemicals and called them endorphins.

Acupuncture is thought to ease pain by activating the brain's own pain-relieving endorphin system, and the system is probably responsible for the 'placebo effect' – the pain relief that one in three people experiences when given a dummy pill which does not actually contain a pain reliever.

We've also learned that other pain relievers like aspirin don't act on the brain but inhibit the release of the pain-sensitising prostaglandins – a discovery which led to the production of a new group of drugs of which ibuprofen is still the only one licensed for sale in Britain without need of a doctor's prescription.

the new techniques but by an understanding by doctors that the techniques must be tailored to the needs of the individual. That is why, if you are threatened by severe pain, you can now be referred, under the NHS, to a specialist pain clinic.

It's sad that medicine's achievements in the control of pain are not more widely known because they have removed one of the great fears that people have about illness. All those diseases traditionally associated with suffering and pain have had their sting removed and the most significant advance in medical care that I have seen in my lifetime has been the development of hospices – institutions dedicated not to curing illness but to taking the pain, and the fear, out of dying.

The skills of hospice doctors and nurses are now so refined that they can give drugs in just the right measure and at just the right times to relieve pain without 'drugging' the senses.

The British actress Sheila Hancock has written a moving account of the way her husband who was dying of cancer spent his last months on this earth free from pain and how, on the evening before he died, they went out together from the hospice to go to dinner and the theatre.

A HEALTHY STYLE OF LIVING

Sense and Nonsense about Diet

What your diet can do to you

The argument about what constitutes a healthy diet is over. A few people with vested interests would like to keep it going but even they are now losing heart because the nutritional experts, while disagreeing about some of the details, have reached agreement about the fundamentals.

In the past, ideas about diet were based on traditional folklore which had never been subjected to scientific scrutiny.

Today's views on what our diet can and cannot do for us are based on evidence accumulated from a wide variety of nutritional studies conducted over the past twenty years: studies of apparent links between diet and health in different parts of the world, investigations of what sorts of foods the human body seems to have been designed to use, studies of the effects of diet on animal and human biochemistry.

As evidence from these studies has accumulated, a nutritional consensus has evolved on what constitutes a healthy diet – one which not only accords with our nutritional needs but also lowers our risk of getting heart disease and cancer, and of becoming overweight.

Scientists still argue about the meaning of some of the evidence but the consensus suggests three simple ways in which we who live in the West can protect our health by changing the balance of our diet:

The three key recommendations

- eat less saturated fat which translates as eat less animal fat

- eat less of the processed calorie-dense foods which allow you to consume large amounts of refined sugar and fat before you feel 'full'

- eat more fibre

The cost benefits

Members of communities which eat the sort of diet those changes would produce are much less liable to suffer from:

- heart disease
- diabetes
- bowel cancer
- other bowel diseases like appendicitis and diverticulitis

- gall bladder disease
- tooth decay
- hiatus hernia
- haemorrhoids
- varicose veins

What you can do to your diet

Less animal fat

If you eat less animal fat, you will lower your risk of heart disease.

Eating less animal fat doesn't mean just eating less fatty meat. Most of our fat intake comes from dairy products. So less animal fat means cutting your consumption of full-cream milk, butter, cream, and fatty cheeses.

Try semi-skimmed milk instead of silver top. I find it hard to tell the difference. Even better, try skimmed milk. You may detect a difference but many who do don't mind it. If you want to eat less butter, experiment with low fat spreads. You may be pleasantly surprised. And don't forget that foods like cakes and biscuits contain lots of hidden fat.

A growing number of nutritionists, though not all, claim you can lower your risk of heart disease by replacing some of the animal fat in your diet with polyunsaturated fat such as that found in sunflower, safflower, maize, and fish.

I'm one of those persuaded by the evidence.

Two years ago, I started to use a polyunsaturated margarine instead of butter on my bread. It took me only a day or two to get used to it and now I actually prefer it. I'm making no sacrifice and I'm pretty sure I'm doing myself some good.

Less sugar, more fibre

Increasing the fibre in your diet will help you lower your risk of bowel cancer, gall bladder disease, and lesser afflictions like haemorrhoids and varicose veins.

Keeping the sugar content of your diet under control will protect you from becoming overweight.

Obesity carries an increased risk of heart disease, and over-weight people live shorter lives and suffer more illness.

You won't have to work hard at cutting the sugar in your diet if you eat it in its natural unrefined form, and the easy way to get the balance of fibre and sugar right is to consider them together.

Carbohydrates, once the villains of the 'slimming diet', are now seen as the key to healthy eating. They are essentially sugars and starches which come almost exclusively from plants in which they are encased within the fibre of the plant's supporting structure. The healthy way to eat them is with their encasing fibre.

Sugar which has been refined out of plants – separated from the fibre – can supply the energy our bodies need but that is all it does supply.

Unrefined sources of carbohydrates – cereals, pulses, potatoes, and roots like cassava – supply not just energy but fibre. And, because they are more filling, they make it less easy for us to consume the excess calories that lead to obesity. It's all too easy to swallow those extra, fattening, calories when we take the less bulky refined sugar that is added to sweetmeats, confectionery and sauces.

How to eat healthily: practical advice

Healthy eating is not a matter of dieting but of balancing. If you get the fat right – not too much – and the carbohydrate right – trying to take most of it in an unrefined form – you will probably get the calories right too.

If you must, you can even eat 'junk food', as long as you don't eat only 'junk'. Junk's drawback is the large amounts of sugars and fat it packs into each mouthful so that, when you try to balance your diet, you have little room for other foods you enjoy.

You can also eat 'convenience foods' though again you have to balance convenience against content. Many contain so much unneeded fat and sugar that they too leave little room for the things that you do need. But shop around. Some food manufacturers and retailers are beginning to respond to pressure from consumers and are producing foods that are both convenient and healthy.

Nutritionists have made other suggestions – that we eat less salt (see page 113, *What should we do about salt?*), for instance – but balancing our consumption of fat, sugar, and fibre is seen as our most urgent need.

Strategy

Why not tackle this business of healthy eating the way you'd tackle any management problem?

The objective is to eliminate unnecessary risks to your health. The methods are outlined above.

But before you settle for a plan let me give you two pieces of advice that might affect your strategy:

- **Strategic rule one: don't go on a diet**
  One of the most formidable barriers to healthy eating is semantic. Many of us think of 'going on a diet' as some sort of punishment for original sin. To redeem inherent naughtiness, we have to give up one of life's great pleasures.

  'Going on a diet' also implies a temporary change; if you go on it, you can come off it. The enjoyable way to eat healthily is to make a permanent change in your pattern of everyday eating.

The good news to emerge from today's nutritional consensus is that for most of us the change in pattern doesn't need to be dramatic but is really just a matter of getting the balance of our eating right.

The even better news is that healthy eating is quite consistent with being a gourmet

- **Strategic rule two: don't become a faddist**
  Do remember that, if you want to eat healthy food, you don't have to become a crank. Quite the opposite. You just have to try to get more pleasure out of eating.

  You can do that by choosing foods you enjoy eating and which fit your balanced diet: more vegetables (those old villains potatoes are now persona grata), more wholegrain products, more fruit as fruit rather than as pie filling, more lean meat, poultry, and fish; more grilling, broiling, and rotisserie, less frying and stewing; food served up crisply as what it is and not buried beneath heavy, rich sauces; mediterranean cuisine, oriental cuisine, nouvelle cuisine . . .

With those guidelines even a dedicated hedonist can discover that the whole idea of being healthy is suddenly attractive.

It's also much easier than it was just two years ago. Enterprising manufacturers are now producing new foods, and reintroducing old ones, to meet our nutritional needs. Grocery stores are responding to the new demands. Chefs and restaurateurs are beginning to recognise the needs of business executives who want to eat healthily.

So let's look at the sort of tactics that might work for you.

Tactics

Useful habits to acquire

- if you like milk in your tea or coffee, use semi-skimmed

- if you like sweet tea or coffee, use saccharin instead of sugar

- switch to wholemeal bread

- eat rice and pasta more often

- if you like cheese, eat low fat cheeses like cottage cheese and curd cheese, or medium fat cheeses like Brie, Camembert and Edam

- cut back on high fat cheeses like Cheddar, Danish Blue, Stilton, and Lymeswold

- if you like butter, try low fat spread or a polyunsaturated margarine. Stick with the margarine for a few days before deciding that it's not for you. It takes time to alter an habituated taste

- eat thicker slices of bread with a thinner layer of 'spread'

- try using yoghurt instead of cream (but be sure that it is labelled 'low fat')

- cut the fat off your meat

- avoid dishes made from mince which you haven't made for yourself. Mince can have a very high fat content

- if you like sausages, eat only those labelled 'low fat'

- if you eat burgers, grill them and eat them with high fibre foods like wholemeal bread or potatoes

- avoid ready-made meat pies which can contain lots of fat

- avoid nibbling at 'snacks' like packets of crisps which provide you with calories you don't need without the fibre that you do

- use sunflower or olive oil for cooking rather than animal fat

Meals you don't have to eat

Do you eat breakfast out of habit? A lot of successful and energetic people manage happily without a large cooked breakfast.

Why not save the 'traditional British breakfast' for an occasional treat – maybe when you're staying in an hotel. On other days try breakfasting on cereal or muesli and some wholemeal toast and fresh fruit.

Give it a go for a few days at least before dismissing it. If some days you feel like a more substantial breakfast, have a kipper, or even two, instead of a traditional fry-up.

Meals you do have to eat

Your least escapable meals are probably business lunches and dinners. They can be a threat to healthy eating habits. But the threat can be averted.

Where to go

If you have the clout, choose the restaurant. If you haven't the clout, try to influence the choice.

The restaurants to go for are Chinese, Italian, other restaurants serving mediterranean cuisine, and French restaurants which serve nouvelle cuisine rather than traditional bourgeois French.

Anton Mosimann, *maître chef* at the Dorchester, has devised 'Cuisine Naturelle' which eschews butter, cream and alcohol and is sparing with salt and sugar. Other hotels and restaurants in growing numbers are ministering to their business clients' wish for healthier meals:

- luxury hotels like London's Inn on the Park now offer an 'alternative menu'

- Hyatt hotels offer a selection of 'Perfect balance' dishes

- hotels like London's Carlton Tower, the Olympian, and *Le Meridien* Piccadilly set aside part of their health and fitness clubs as a 'Healthy Eaters' restaurant'

- hotel chains like Crest, Sofitel, Trust House Forte, and Marriott offer healthy 'executive breakfasts'

What to choose on the menu

- fish, chicken (remove the skin) rather than red meat

- home made soup rather than pâté

- grilled, poached, steamed or dry sautéd food rather than fried
- liver or kidney, which are not as fatty as other meats
- jacket potatoes rather than *pommes frites*
- crisp, lightly cooked vegetables without cream or cheese sauce
- lean meat from the rotisserie rather than stew
- fresh fruit and low fat cheese rather than creamy dessert
- decaffeinated rather than straight coffee after lunch will lessen your level of unproductive tension during the afternoon; after dinner it will be less likely to cause you a sleepless night

Quick convenient meals and snacks

- choose Chinese takeaway rather than hamburgers
- choose wholemeal sandwiches filled with salad, or fish, or cottage cheese rather than white bread sandwiches filled with processed meat
- drink mineral water – or old-fashioned tap water – rather than branded soft drinks which contain refined sugar
- if you must eat between meals, eat fresh fruit rather than chocolates
- if you are an inveterate nibbler, buy a fruit bowl for your office and, when in need, reach for it
- if you go out for a drink after work, try not to wolf the crisps and salted peanuts. Lots of bars now supply slices of vegetables as 'cocktail snacks'. If the ones you frequent don't, eating an apple before you leave the office will take the edge off the hunger you will be tempted to assuage with crisps

Adopt a business-like approach to diet

Train yourself to think about nutritional value for money in the food you purchase, in a business where the bottom line is yourself:

- how much good does the food you buy do you?

- how easily are you conned by those who stuff their pies with fat because it's cheaper than meat?

A growing bunch of enterprising manufacturers is offering nutritional value for money. The less enterprising still like to pretend that no nutritional consensus has emerged.

Don't be misled by the public relations battle that goes on. You're probably too busy doing your own job to follow the details of arguments about diet. Just as you probably know enough about public relations to understand how the arguments can be distorted.

I repeat what I said on page 105. The argument about what constitutes a healthy diet is over.

Your objective now should be to put the nutritional knowledge that we have to profitable use.

What should we do about salt?

Salt – sodium chloride – is the main source of sodium in our diet and, for fifty years, medical researchers have accumulated evidence that high blood pressure may be linked with sodium intake.

These experimental links raise two questions:

- if we all ate less salt would we lower our risk of getting high blood pressure and therefore our risk of having a heart attack or stroke?

- can people who already have high blood pressure reduce that pressure by eating less salt?

Less salt for us all?
No clear answer comes from the experts because they disagree over the interpretation of the scientific evidence.

The World Health Organisation, and some national nutritional advisory committees, have found the evidence persuasive

A crucial question

One day, out of the blue, I received an invitation to lunch with the group board of a large public company.

The invitation puzzled me. I didn't know any of the directors and, as far as I knew, the company's activities didn't impinge on mine. But being a curious fellow I went along.

By the time we reached the coffee, I was no wiser.

When I'd arrived the chairman had explained that once a month they invited a guest to discuss some aspect of their business. But he left it at that and dropped no hint of what he expected of me.

Come the coffee, he turned to me and said: 'Dr O'Donnell, we hope you will be able to solve a problem which is troubling this company at the highest level.

'Indeed you have it within your power to heal a rift in the board which, if it ever became known outside, could destroy our credibility in the City.'

I felt my throat go dry as he heaped the responsibility upon me. 'The question we would like you to answer is this. When we have lunch in this boardroom, should we or should we not have salt-cellars on the table?'

It was, of course, a sort of joke. But only sort of. Behind the question, it turned out, lay weeks of lunchtime discussion.

Members of that board, like many others, had been confused by conflicting public utterances about dietary salt, and I ended my lunch trying to guide them through the complexities of the evidence before reaching the same conclusions that I do in the section opposite.

When I'd finished and had answered a few questions, my hosts had a quick discussion before reaching a consentient compromise. They would keep the salt-cellars on the table but would put no salt in them.

It seemed a sensible reaction to our present state of knowledge and they told me that the company's success had been built on similar Solomon-like decisions.

I took that with a pinch of salt.

enough to recommend that we restrict the salt in our diet.

The same evidence has failed to convince other reputable scientists, though they accept that eating less salt would do us little harm.

Less salt for people with raised blood pressure?
Here there is similar disagreement over the evidence.

One group of experts quotes scientific studies which seem to show that a moderate restriction of salt – using less salt in cooking, banning the salt-cellar from the table – does actually lower high blood pressure.

A smaller group – but one with equally impressive scientific credentials – claims that the lowering of blood pressure in those studies could have been produced by other dietary changes which occurred at the same time.

They also quote other studies which, though fewer in number, failed to detect any lowering of raised blood pressure in patients who ate less salt.

So what should you do?
Until we get more evidence, or more agreement on the evidence, what you do will depend on the view you take of dietary salt. That is how the scientists themselves behave.

Those who think that a policy of restricting salt is akin to introducing a new drug demand a rigorous evaluation of detailed scientific evidence before making any change.

Those who believe that the amount of salt in our diet has risen so high that restricting it is more akin to removing a toxic agent from our environment say the evidence we already have is enough to suggest a change now, though we should continue investigations until we get a clearer picture.

The second attitude is that taken by the World Health Organisation and the one I recommend.

The evidence that most impresses me is that every doctor I know who himself has high blood pressure now eats less salt, and that many doctor parents now discourage their families, and themselves, from adding salt to their food.

Positive action

- ban salt-cellars from your table
- when they're present on other people's tables, use them only if the food is so tasteless that it's inedible
- when cooking, use no more salt than you need to produce the flavour you want
- cut your consumption of heavily salted foods. No need to avoid them completely. Save those that you like for an occasional treat
- don't use salt substitutes. They could do you more harm than salt

Fish: Britain's forgotten food

One of the lesser quirks of the British is that, though our islands are surrounded by seas richly populated with fish, we eat less seafood than most other nations.

Even more oddly when we travel abroad we enthuse about, and eagerly devour, local seafood in countries which have much shorter coastlines than our own.

Yet we were once great fish eaters and the decline of our fishing industry, thanks largely to wilful neglect, is one of the shameful political tales of post-war Britain. This island race now eats only one eighth as much fish as we eat meat.

History is studded with fanciful claims about the nutritional virtues of fish – when I was a child my mother used to exhort me to eat up my fish because it would give me 'more brains' – but recently substantial scientific reasons have emerged to encourage you to choose fish more often for your executive luncheon.

Fifteen years ago, when the evidence that seemed to link coronary heart disease with a high consumption of fat was beginning to look formidable, one huge flaw in the theory was that Eskimos living in Greenland, who took a staggering 70 per cent of their calorie intake in the form of fat, suffered less heart disease than people who consumed a much lower percentage.

Eat fish and live longer

From 1960 to 1980, a group of researchers at the University of Leiden monitored the diet and the health of 852 middle-aged men living in Zutphen, an old industrial town in the eastern part of the Netherlands.

In 1960 all the men were apparently healthy but, during the following twenty years, seventy-eight of them died from coronary heart disease. When the researchers analysed the statistics, making allowance for other variations in the men's diet, they found that the death rate from coronary heart disease for men who ate no fish was more than twice that for men who ate a moderate amount of fish.

One or two fish dishes a week, they concluded, might help prevent coronary heart disease.

The Dutch study seemed to confirm observations previously made in Japan where the low level of coronary heart disease has been attributed to the high level of fish consumption.

There are also some fascinating variations within Japan.

The country's lowest death rates from coronary heart disease are on the island of Okinawa where the people eat about twice as much fish as their compatriots on the mainland.

And when a group of Japanese researchers studied two villages in Chiba Prefecture, they found that deaths from coronary heart disease were significantly lower in a fishing village than they were in a nearby farming village where the farmers consumed about a third as much fish as the fisherfolk.

Fish is thought to protect the heart by supplying the body with substances which make blood clot more slowly. When Japanese fishermen cut themselves, they bleed for a slightly longer time than other people.

Their less clottable blood is therefore less likely to coagulate in the narrow coronary arteries of the heart and produce the blockage that causes a heart attack.

Since then nutritionists have discovered that the nature of the fat we eat is probably more important than the total amount. The fat linked with heart disease is saturated fat, most commonly found in dairy products and fatty meat; the fat eaten by the Eskimos, who used to live almost entirely on a diet of oily fish, was polyunsaturated fat.

Not only does polyunsaturated fat seem less likely to be associated with heart disease, but the polyunsaturated fats found in fish seem to be positively beneficial to the heart.

The hunt is on to find the reasons why.

A theory that wins much support is that one component of the polyunsaturated fat in fish – it's called EPA – breaks down in our bodies into substances which make our blood less likely to clot in the narrow arteries of the heart.

This theory has led some doctors to recommend regular doses of codliver oil or fish oil capsules – which again conjure up memories of my childhood – as a means of warding off heart disease.

But you'll be even better off consuming the EPA in the original fish . . . and not only because it is more pleasurable.

Though oily fish contains lots of EPA, lean fish contains little.

Yet recent studies have shown that lean fish too can cut the risk of heart disease. It's therefore likely that EPA is not the only fishy ingredient to offer protection.

And fish has other nutritional virtues beyond its heart protecting quality.

The high consumption of saturated fat in Western countries has given fat a bad name but certain sorts of fat are vital to our well being – the fats, for instance, with which we build the cells of our brains and nervous systems.

Fish has proved to be one of the richest sources of those fats – so maybe my mother was on to something after all.

| Positive action |

There's now strong evidence that if you eat fish instead of meat on at least two days a week, you will lower your risk of heart disease:

- don't eat fish smothered under a creamy sauce or have it deep fried in batter – unless it is fried in vegetable oil (as it now is in the best fish and chip shops)

- have your fish grilled, poached, baked, or steamed, and be adventurous in your choice. Fish comes in a great variety of forms and even the worst of cooks have to try really hard to render fish unpalatable

- choose fish you enjoy eating. While you're enjoying yourself, you'll also be doing yourself some good. (Though why exactly you are doing yourself good may take a few more years to discover)

There's a sad footnote to this unfinished story.

Most of the Greenland Eskimos, whose freedom from heart disease set the scientists off on their promising trail, have now changed to a Westernised diet. And with our diet they have also acquired our pattern of disease.

The slimming game

This is one of Britain's most popular indoor sports and supports a fair sized industry which produces diet magazines and newspapers, diet books, diet foods, saunas, steam baths, exercise machinery, self-help groups, and a multitude of strange devices. The industry serves an eager market.

Every year one in three British adults tries to lose weight. The fact that this figure stays constant suggests that few of the diets and other slimming aids have much effect.

That's no great surprise because most people have no idea that if they want to lose a substantial amount of weight, the time they need to stay on a restricted diet has to be measured in years rather than months.

Most believe, quite wrongly, that once they've got their weight down to the level they desire, they can give up the diet, return to their former lifestyle, yet still stay at their new weight.

Being overweight does carry penalties. It increases the risk of heart, chest, and gall bladder disease, and of some forms of arthritis and cancer.

If you want to know if you are running that risk, plot your position on the following chart:

WEIGHT-CHECK CHART

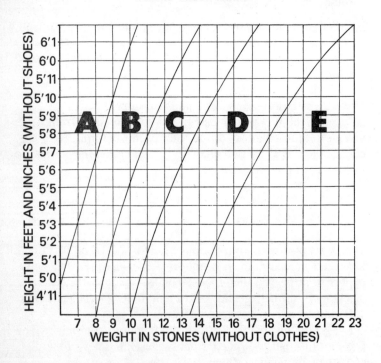

Zone A   You are underweight. It might be a good idea to have a medical check-up or, at least, a word with your doctor

Zone B   This is the healthiest zone to occupy

Zone C   You are overweight. Nothing to worry about. But don't get any fatter

Zone D   You are too fat. You are running a risk of ill-health unless you lose weight

Zone E   You are dangerously fat. You should seek medical advice about getting your weight down – and seek it urgently

If you are in Zone E, you really should seek medical advice. In Zone D you should try to move yourself to Zone B. In Zone C, you don't need to worry, but you'd probably feel fitter if you crossed the border into Zone B. The best way to move to a healthier zone is not to go on a temporary slimming kick but to try to change your behaviour permanently. The aim is take in less energy, burn off more, or do both.

Burning more energy sounds a logical way of losing weight but nutritional research has shown it is not very efficient: you have to use up a lot of energy to lose very little weight. Still, some people do find that regular exercise helps keep their weight under control. (See page 126, *Can exercise help you lose weight?*) It's worth a trial because it could work for you.

Most people, however, think of losing weight in terms of 'slimming' which means cutting down their energy intake by going on a diet. I've described on page 108 that the main snag about going on a diet is that 'going on' implies 'coming off' – so, from the beginning, there's an implication that the change of diet is temporary.

And while a diet which cuts your energy intake may help you to get yourself literally into shape, once the diet is over you're likely to drift back into the less desirable zones of the chart. To change your chart zone permanently you need to change the balance of your diet permanently by eating less fat, less refined sugar, more fibre.

Yet there are times when a burst of 'slimming' seems the right response. One is when you try on spring or summer clothes and find they seem to have shrunk in the waistband and under the armpits since you wore them last year.

Those extra pounds you acquired during the winter may weigh heavily upon your mind and, if you feel a desperate need to get rid of them, there's no harm in going on a diet that cuts down your calorie (i.e. energy) intake.

A short punishing 'diet' will also satisfy the feeling, which many of us share, that health can come only out of suffering. An American woman who survived a serious car accident after a dinner party told her doctor: 'As the truck came at me all that went through my head was that, if I'm going to get killed, what a fool I was to pass up the dessert.'

If you settle for a burst of slimming, you'll have little trouble finding a diet. In spring and early summer, as people contemplate the inflated silhouettes of winter, slimming diets burst forth in magazines and newspapers with the same profligacy as spring bulbs and flowering shrubs.

The diets come in two main varieties, the low carbohydrate and the calorie counting.

I'm not mad about the low carbohydrate approach (and its close cousin, the 'eat as much fat as you like' diet) because it involves cutting down on healthy foods like bread and potatoes where the complex carbohydrates are integrated with their natural fibre, and because it tilts the balance of fat in the diet in the direction which we now know to be unhealthy.

If you must go on a diet, I recommend you go on a calorie counting diet. This means setting yourself a target of calories per day and then, using a chart which gives the caloric value of foods, working out a diet which falls within your limit.

If you do this and also choose foods which follow the guidelines described on pages 105–7, you don't have to abandon the healthy balance of your normal diet.

If you do decide to count the calories, you'll find it rewarding to set the upper limit at a level which is severe enough not just to produce joy on the weighing scales but to inspire a smug feeling that you are suffering in a good cause.

Then, one day when the suffering is at its most intense, give a thought to the idea of escaping the need for an annual slimming penance by making a more lasting change to your lifestyle. Most people find the permanent change much more rewarding than the penance, and certainly much more enjoyable.

A word of warning. Don't punish yourself too severely. There's been a recent fashion for very low calorie diets which involve giving up normal food and taking nutritionally balanced substitutes.

These diets can get rid of weight quickly but their long term efficacy is very much in doubt. Many who lose weight while on the diet get it back quickly when they go back to normal food.

Very low calorie diets are not a good idea for those who wish to move out of Zones C and D. Their prolonged use may lead to loss not just of fat but of lean muscle tissue, which is the tissue that burns up energy. The dieters can end up losing some of their capacity to burn off calories which means that in future they will have to store those calories as fat and, although the initial weight loss may seem spectacular, they will find it more difficult to keep their weight at a lower level.

If you go on a diet you must be prepared to lose weight gradually. The first weight to go will be water and this can return as quickly as it was lost. After the water has gone, rapid weight loss can be achieved only at the expense of lean tissue and the more rapid the weight loss, the greater will be the proportion of lean tissue.

If, after the initial water loss, you are losing more than one or two pounds a week, you are almost certainly losing non-fat tissue and you could be damaging your health.

Positive action

The best way to keep your weight under control is not to go on an occasional 'diet' but to make a permanent change in your regular eating habits. But first you may need to get your weight down:

- set yourself a target weight and then reduce the amount of fat you eat and take some moderate regular exercise

- cutting down on refined sugar and alcohol will also help

- once you've got down to your target weight, you can eat more. But don't go back to fatty food and do keep an eye on the scales

- if you do decide to go on a diet, choose a calorie counting diet and be prepared to lose weight gradually. Losing body fat takes time

- don't use a very low calorie diet, unless advised to by a doctor. The weight you lose may soon return and you may find it more difficult to keep your weight at a lower level

Sense and Nonsense about Exercise

Health or fashion?

Future historians in search of symbols of our times may well cite our vigorous promotion of physical activity as a source of health. Its promotion, often appropriately breathless, has at times owed less to reason than to enthusiasm, fantasy, and wish fulfilment. No public park now seems complete without its posse of joggers, no city can claim to be a major one unless it has an annual marathon.

Is this resurgence of faith in the health-giving properties of exercise merely a cult or is it backed by scientific evidence? Scientific knowledge of the effects of exercise has failed to keep pace with the enthusiasm of many of the participants and while positivists can use what evidence we have to rally the faithful, negativists have also used it to show that exercise brings few health benefits and can indeed be dangerous.

Disputes about the evidence have grown more raucous since that day in August 1984 when Jim Fixx, the joggers' guru, dropped dead while at his exercise. When the news got out, the negativists won a lot of converts. How stands the argument now?

I regard myself as a neutral in the debate and the conclusions presented in this chapter are those I have reached after casting what I hope is a sceptical eye at the evidence.

What can exercise do for you?

- **Regular endurance exercise helps reduce the risk of heart attacks**
  Two scientifically impeccable studies of the habits of London

civil servants and of middle aged employees at Stanford University in California showed that thirty to forty-five minutes spent each week on endurance exercise (see page 128) which was energetic enough to generate a mild sweat and cause breathlessness could dramatically reduce the risk of heart attacks.

Scientists have yet to define exactly why it should. They've produced convincing theories but still lack the evidence needed to sustain them.

- **Regular exercise helps keep muscles and joints in working order**
Regular exercise has parallels with regular car maintenance. Not only does it keep the moving parts in working order but it prevents the decline in strength, suppleness and stamina which can come with age but which is not, as many people think, inevitable.

Scientists have validated an observation which most of us have made for ourselves. We know that if we repeat the same physical activity daily, we can, after a time, complete it without growing as hot and breathless as we did at our first attempt.

Measurement of oxygen uptake and of changes in body chemistry have now shown that repetition – 'training' – literally does make our hearts and muscles work more efficiently and that this effect works at all ages. Middle-aged and elderly people adapt to training in the same way, if not at the same speed, as do young adults.

- **Exercise keeps the whole body active**
People who 'maintain' their bodies can indulge in a far wider range of physical activities than those who don't, and their bodies can cope with sudden stresses which might otherwise injure them, like having to run for a bus, carry a heavy package, or walk across country or along deserted roads in search of help when the car breaks down.

- **Exercise can relieve tension and anxiety**
But it has to be exercise you enjoy taking, not exercise you take to satisfy an obsession. Exercise you enjoy taking

can clear your mind of worries that nag at it, produce a sense of well being, and help you to sleep more soundly and refreshingly.

• **Exercise can make you feel good**
The best reason of all for taking exercise. If you enjoy it, you will also enjoy the feeling of fitness it produces.

Exercise does not have to be competitive. The best reasons for taking regular exercise have less to do with athletic machismo than with maintaining your body's strength, stamina and suppleness.

Can exercise help you lose weight?

I'm as yet more intrigued than convinced by evidence that regular exercise may help keep people's weight down.

On the face of it, exercise would seem a poor way to lose weight because you need to engage in so much activity to 'burn off' so few calories.

Yet some researchers have shown that sustained exercise can increase oxygen consumption – used in burning off calories – for more than 24 hours after the exercise ceases and may dramatically increase oxygen consumption after subsequent meals, which suggests that the calories taken in with the meal are being rapidly burned off.

This has led to the suggestion that regular sustained aerobic exercise – endurance rather than 'sprint' exercise – can cause a permanent increase in the rate at which the body uses energy, as if it had been refitted with an engine hungrier for fuel.

Regular aerobic exercise, goes the theory, if it is combined with a well-balanced diet, will help people not just to lose weight but to keep their weight at a lower level.

A persuasive advocate of this theory is Geoffrey Cannon, co-author of *Dieting Makes You Fat* (Sphere) who once calculated that during his thirties, when he fought a running battle with his weight by dieting, he had shed some fourteen stone and, if he'd regained none of it, he'd have entered his forties weighing minus one and a half stone.

How dieting can make you fat: the theory

The rationale of losing weight by dieting is that when energy intake is lower than energy expenditure, the body will make up the deficit by burning off the excess fat it has laid down to meet just such a need.

In practice, much of the weight lost when someone first goes on a low calorie diet is not fat. The body draws first on a more immediate energy source: glycogen, a carbohydrate stored in watery solution in the muscles and liver.

Only after the body has bridged the energy gap by burning up glycogen will it start to lose fat and muscle and, when it does, an obese and relatively inactive person will lose more muscle than a slim and active person.

Indeed, physical activity during a diet can encourage the loss of more fat and less muscle.

People prepared to follow a low calorie diet for a long time will not regain the weight they initially lost, which was made up of water, glycogen, fat and muscle.

Less heroic folk, once they achieve a reasonable weight, tend to strut around proudly for a while in clothes that had ceased to fit them, then return quietly to their previous eating habits. When they do, there's one way in which they are worse off than they were. They replace the lost glycogen and the lost fat but they will not replace the lost muscle. So they increase the proportion of 'flab' in their bodies.

The body can also respond to the energy deprivation imposed by a diet by lowering the rate at which it uses energy – its metabolic rate.

This lowering may be the cause of some of the symptoms experienced by dieters or noticed by people around them: irritability, depression, and a general 'slowing down' that involves spells of sleepiness or of aimless inactivity.

Though scientists still argue over the physiological details on which this theory is based, it has practical virtues: it seems to work for a lot of people and does none of them any harm.

Now, he says, exercise allows him to keep it under control without getting involved in the depressing cycle of heroic dieting followed by shameful backsliding.

Many nutritionists claim there's little evidence to support the theory that regular exercise can permanently increase the rate at which the body uses energy.

Cannon counters by claiming that his critics have done the wrong experiments, often taking a group of relatively unfit people and training them casually for a few weeks. He would like them to repeat their measurements on a group of volunteers who would follow a carefully monitored exercise programme for at least a year.

He also quotes back evidence that aerobic exercise which is vigorous enough to more than double the heart rate and which continues for at least twenty minutes, does produce an increase in metabolic rate (the rate at which the body consumes energy) which can persist for several hours.

On the eve of his fortieth birthday, Cannon took up jogging and, as the months went by, discovered he had managed to escape from the diet/backsliding cycle. He claims he has since found many overweight people like himself who started running, lost weight, and now eat and drink what they like without having to fear the bathroom scales.

I'm happy, with one proviso, to recommend a Cannon-style routine of regular exercise on the pragmatic grounds that it seems to help a lot of people to keep their weight down.

My only proviso is that you should enjoy the exercise.

What sort of exercise is healthy?

Let's start with a few definitions:

Aerobic exercise is endurance exercise which calls more on stamina than on short explosive bursts of activity. It can lower the risk of heart attack if it is taken regularly – for at least thirty to forty-five minutes per week – at a level which makes the heart beat faster and causes some breathlessness.

Don't forget that jogging and distance running are not the only forms of aerobic exercise. Tennis, cycling (including riding an exercise bicycle), swimming, even vigorous walking, are equally effective and may appeal to you more.

Anaerobic exercise is more an explosive 'sprint' form of exercise than a stamina one. Typical examples are squash, athletic field events and sprinting.

Many sports, like tennis and football, involve a mixture of aerobic and anaerobic exercise. The adjectives refer to the mechanism by which energy is produced in the muscles and that becomes anaerobic only when the muscles are called on for sudden explosive activity. So, depending on how they play the game, you could say that some people's football is more aerobic than others'.

Healthy exercise, in my book, is any exercise you enjoy taking.

Unhealthy exercise is exercise you don't enjoy yet persist with in the hope that it might be 'doing you good'. Martyrdom is not an essential prerequisite of health.

Types of exercise

The scientific case for the benefits of *vigorous* exercise remains largely unproven and a vast amount of research still needs to be done.

Clearly it is healthy if it helps those who are physically fit to engage in activities from which they draw rewards: a sense of achievement, a chance to indulge their competitiveness, to make new friends, broaden their horizons, and have fun.

It is less healthy when it is indulged in by people who have not trained themselves to the necessary fitness and who, if they are middle-aged, may overtax their bodies to a dangerous extent.

The case for *less vigorous* exercise is clearer. We now know that regular exercise that makes us breathless and makes us sweat a bit *can* cut our risk of a heart attack.

We also know that if exercise is to be beneficial it has to be a lifelong activity. University athletes who later give up exercise seem to run a greater risk of heart disease than those who have never been athletic.

We still don't know the best form of exercise for people to continue with after they give up the vigorous athletic activities of youth, but most of the evidence of benefit comes from studies of people who walked a lot, used stairs instead of lifts, or dug their gardens regularly.

As yet there is no unassailable evidence that runners, short distance or marathon distance, give their hearts any more protection than they would get from other regular but less rigorous aerobic exercise. But then people have other good reasons for running, such as enjoying it or because it makes them *feel* better.

How dangerous is exercise?

The question has been asked more insistently since Jim Fixx dropped dead while jogging. That was an unusual incident because the most serious risks of exercise – heart attacks and disordered rhythm of the heart – are associated with sudden and unaccustomed exercise.

Jim Fixx seems, from published accounts, to have been a victim not of exercise but of an obsession to push himself constantly beyond the limits which his body tried to impose on him.

Yet the question remains. Do men and women who engage in rigorous exercise – particularly in middle-age – run an increased risk of sudden death?

The answer seems to depend on the form of exercise. The evidence suggests that aerobic exercise does not increase the risk while anaerobic exercise does increase it, though not dramatically.

So the message to the middle-aged is that, if they want to take up exercise after a long spell of inactivity, they should take up aerobic exercise and work their way into it gradually. Squash is more hazardous for those who take it up late or who play only occasionally in middle age than for those who have played regularly, say at least three times a week, since they were young.

It is a dangerous game for 'macho' competitors over the age of forty who play only occasionally.

Taking up exercise in middle age and beyond

You don't have to give up competitive games as you grow older. My late and much lamented friend George Mikes played tennis every week up to the seventy-sixth and last year of his life and was, I'm told, a difficult man to beat.

People like George are the reason why no one can set an age at which people should give up vigorous physical activity. And he was not alone. Borotra played at Wimbledon at the age of seventy-three and every sport can produce its heroes who go on playing to a grand old age.

These people cope with the exertion comfortably because they have exercised regularly, without break, right through their adult lives. Many a middle-aged businessman who reads about them, or sees them on a television screen as he props his paunch against the club bar, wishes he could emulate them. How dangerous is it for him to try?

If he already takes regular vigorous exercise – vigorous means jogging rather than golf – he has no problem. It is safe for him to continue for as long as he wants, provided the exercise does not cause him too much distress. Judging what is too much is a matter of common sense rather than of medical expertise.

More difficult is the decision facing the man, or woman, who has not taken any vigorous exercise for years but would now like to start again. Once you get into your late thirties and beyond, nursing your body back to some sort of physical fitness is a tedious business. It needs more patience than vigour.

I remember, at about that age, having a sudden desire to become physically fitter. I started on the Canadian Air Force physical fitness programme (published still by Penguin) but found that I was allowed to do so little in the early weeks that I grew bored and gave up before I reached the more interesting exercises.

Sadly, there are no short cuts. Overweight executives who

want to take up jogging should not start until they have slowly edged their way towards fitness by doing graduated exercise, preferably under professional supervision in a gym. There they can work their way through a progressive series of activities planned for them by qualified trainers who will monitor their pulse rates and their pulse recovery times.

The only alternative is to exercise literally by the book, using the Canadian Air Force programme or one of the many other published texts. This really is a poor alternative and, these days, most office blocks have a friendly neighbourhood gym or fitness centre.

A middle-aged return to exercise should not be an isolated gesture. It must be part of a change of lifestyle which includes other healthy moves like getting your weight down, cutting out cigarettes, maybe altering your drinking habits. Then, if your doctor gives you an all clear after a physical examination, a return to regular exercise can produce not just physical fitness but a rewarding feeling of well-being.

If you want to get fit for a particular sport like tennis or skiing or the sport of the moment, marathon running, seek the advice of a doctor who himself or herself takes part in the sport.

Other doctors will give you generalised advice. The doctor who knows the sport through personal experience will give you the detailed advice you need: specific exercises, when to do them, how to progress them, and – most important of all – how not to do them.

Thanks to the recherché attitude my profession has to advertising, the only way to find a knowledgeable doctor is to ask around. Most sports involve your joining a club and that's the place to do the asking. The last person I advised to do that asked someone he met in the bar and found he was talking to a doctor.

Remember too that even if you do everything right, starting slowly and progressing gradually until you get yourself as fit as you can, sports injuries come more easily to those who have waved goodbye to youth. Muscles pull and ligaments strain more easily. They also take longer to heal.

When I was working as a junior doctor in a hospital, one of our senior surgeons was a physical fitness fanatic. His junior had to

Athletic ambition in middle age

One month before my forty-ninth birthday, I was on holiday with my family. Over breakfast, my teenage daughter bragged about her tennis and I challenged her to a match.

In my youth I'd been a handy player and that morning, once I'd got my limbs loose and my eye in, half-remembered skills began to flow into my racket.

I tried not to run around the court too much and, thanks mainly to low cunning, managed to win. I retired to the shower short of puff but full of pride.

That evening I walked into the hotel dining room giving a fair imitation of Quasimodo in *The Hunchback of Notre Dame*. Every muscle I'd learned about in medical school was painful and inflexible. I even ached in muscles I never knew I had.

It was a neat cumuppence.

For years I'd been telling patients that, as they grew older, they needed to ease themselves gently into new physical activity. Yet the excitement of the moment had driven all thought of my own advice from my mind. Like everybody else, I had been delighted to discover that some of the old skills had been stored away in some dusty corner of my brain.

And, like everybody else, I had found out too late that a middle-aged body driven to violent exercise flatters only to deceive. My only consolation was that the game hadn't provoked a heart attack.

meet him at 7 am every morning on the squash court and give him a vigorous game before going off to operate. The surgeon was in his early sixties and played with fierce enthusiasm. (Rumour had it that the way to get a good reference was to give him a good competitive game but never actually beat him.)

That man was as fit as man can be, but one morning he dashed across the court no more vigorously than usual and ruptured his Achilles tendon. We all tried not to laugh too loudly when we heard the news.

Yet, even with his specialised knowledge, he couldn't accept that this was the sort of failure you must expect in a sixty year old mechanism. He attributed it to lack of fitness and his next junior, poor chap, had to join him in a weight training programme.

If you'd like to get out of your office chair and become physically active again, don't feel you have to take up the fashionable jog or return to the team games you once enjoyed. Activities like hill-walking or sailing offer healthy exercise and are easier to keep up as you grow older. They will keep your muscles and joints in working order and can bring greater intellectual rewards than more vigorous, and accident-prone, team games.

Having settled for a form of exercise you enjoy, try to avoid making it competitive – a severe act of self-denial, I know, for many a business executive. Enjoy the activity for its own sake and try not to become obsessed with it. If there are days when you don't feel like taking exercise, then give yourself a break. It's not a good idea, for instance, to take vigorous exercise if you're suffering from a virus infection.

Whatever you do, don't force yourself into exercise you don't enjoy because you think it is making you healthy.

Some sensible precautions

A few simple precautions can reduce the risks of exercise:

- don't indulge in vigorous outdoor exercise in very hot or very cold weather or within two hours of a heavy meal

- don't plunge straight into vigorous exercise without first warming up

- allow time for a spell of 'cooling down' relaxation after the exercise

- check on the credentials of anyone who purports to supervise your exercise, be they 'trainer', gymnasium coach, or aerobic dance leader. Ask to see their qualifications. They should at least have a certificate from a recognised training course. If you're uncertain of the status of the certificate, check with the

Citizens' Advice Bureau. Unqualified teachers – and there are a lot of them about – can do you more harm than good

- if your approach is not masochistic but a simple search for a feeling of 'fitness', stop the exercise if it starts to hurt

Three words of warning to the lonely long distance runner

The 'exercise boom' has encouraged lots of people who have led sedentary lives for years to take up jogging and long distance running. Many have become members of clubs or learned the 'dos and don'ts' from one of the books of instruction their sport has spawned. They will understand the need for carefully regulated training and will have learned from dedicated athletes how to avoid some of the hazards of their sport.

People who take up running at a less intense level, very often on their own, are so beguiled by it that their enthusiasm carries them away and they stretch themselves physically before they're really prepared. Over the past decade, doctors have defined three hazards which are often unrecognised by long distance runners whose enthusiasm for their sport exceeds their knowledge of it:

- hypoglycemia – low blood sugar

- hyperthermia – overheating

- dehydration

- **Hypoglycemia**
  Prolonged muscle activity may use up all the body's stores of glucose. Television viewers have seen the effects of the resultant low blood sugar in marathon runners who enter the stadium at the end of their race lurching from side to side and making grossly uncoordinated efforts to reach the finishing line. They look dangerously ill yet an intravenous dose of glucose can produce a rapid recovery.

  You can prevent hypoglycemia by sucking glucose sweets or tablets to replace the glucose fuel that your muscles are burning up. (Just as, when the weather is hot, salt tablets can replace the salt lost in sweat and so ward off the muscle weariness and cramps that come with salt depletion.)

• Hyperthermia and Dehydration

Sustained exercise dramatically increases the body's production of heat which it tries to lose by increasing the blood flow through the skin and by producing sweat which needs heat to evaporate it. A runner may lose several litres of sweat during a marathon yet if the day is hot, and humid enough to slow the vaporisation of sweat, the heat loss may be inadequate and the body's internal temperature will rise.

You can reduce the risk of hyperthermia and dehydration by drinking water before and during a race and by repeatedly dousing your body, vest, and shorts with water to encourage cooling evaporation.

A simple test for hyperthermia is to feel the skin at the top of your chest. If it is hot and dry, you should slow and drink some water as soon as possible.

The test is not wholly reliable and anyone who feels ill when running on a hot humid day should stop and seek medical advice.

A cautionary tale for all who exercise

Jim Smith built his success in business on the same qualities that had made him a successful sportsman. He was highly competitive, worked long energetic hours and, when the going got tough, revealed that an uncompromising edge lay not too deep beneath his genial exterior.

He collected business rewards as inevitably as he had once collected university sporting trophies.

At work, he demanded high standards from everybody and, as a hard but fair taskmaster, ran a string of successful operations. Yet he never quite commanded the loyalty of those who worked for him. His obsessional nature made it difficult for him to inspire others.

Jim trained as hard to keep himself fit for business as he had once trained himself to keep himself fit for sport. He started each day with an hour of jogging; he avoided business lunches and went instead to a gym; in the evenings and at weekends, his juniors were expected to make themselves available for sporting demolition on squash or tennis court. Four times a year he ran a full length marathon.

Five years ago, when he was still in his late thirties, his career started to crumble. He was still fiercely competitive but his work began to lose the qualities that had distinguished it: thorough research, attention to detail, a determination to beat the opposition through sheer hard work.

The more cynical and less energetic readers of this page will already have decided he was exhausted by all that exercise. The truth is slightly odder.

Jim had developed a pathological obsession with the notion of 'keeping fit'. It grew to dominate his life and, as training and exercise consumed more and more hours of each day, he had to relegate his work to second place. As others grow addicted to drugs, Jim had grown addicted to 'fitness'.

That form of addiction can include a physical element. When long distance runners break through the 'pain barrier' they can experience an enjoyable sensation of well-being produced by chemicals which their muscles release into their blood and which stimulate 'pleasure centres' in the brain.

They can also grow 'addicted' to the commendable idea of improving their performance, of setting higher standards and of achieving them. While that is an 'addiction' which enriches, the enrichment can all too easily turn into destructiveness. This was what happened with Jim Smith's addiction. His obsession with 'fitness' slowly took over his life to the exclusion of everything else.

Many successful people will recognise the obsession because they have been tempted by it. Most manage to reject the temptation but what can be done for those who succumb?

Jim Smith was lucky to have a doctor whom he trusted, whose advice he was prepared to follow, and who was there to support him when things threatened to go wrong.

His doctor first advised him to change his job so that he could start in a new place with a new set of values. He also encouraged Jim to cultivate what he called 'a few redeeming defects'.

He didn't discourage him from seeking perfection in everything he did. That would have hobbled the valuable drive he brought to his work. But he did encourage him not to grow too desperate when perfection eluded him, and persuaded him to explore some pleasures of life he could share with other people.

The treatment worked and Jim's second business venture is now more successful than his first could ever have hoped to be.

He is also a happier, and healthier, man.

The Trouble with Booze

Counting the cost

Over the past twenty years the incidence of alcohol abuse in Britain has doubled and many of us have grown impervious to the statistics:

- some three million people in Britain suffer the catastrophic medical and social effects of alcohol abuse.
- one in six accident and emergency cases treated in British hospitals is alcohol-related. That's over two million people a year or one every fifteen seconds.
- government research indicates that industry loses between eight million and fourteen million days a year because of absenteeism following heavy drinking.
- an 'extremely conservative' estimate by York University economists of the financial cost – losses to industry, demands on health services and police, damage to property, and so on – suggests it is at least two billion pounds a year.

These are just numbers that a news-reader reels off in the background while we're busy ordering another round. No one wants to be a killjoy. And plenty of people are eager to advise us not to worry. Have another drink and cheer yourself up.

A couple of nights I spent as an observer in a hospital emergency department taught me not to equate alcohol abuse with 'alcoholism'. It has some more blatant manifestations, like domestic violence and football hooliganism.

It also has some that are less blatant, but no less pernicious,

like the erosion of efficiency in young adults setting out to build a
future in the world of business – an erosion that too often brings a
catastrophic early end to a promising career.

Until I looked at the figures, and at the victims, I wasn't
overconcerned about youthful drunkenness. Young people have
always enjoyed drinking too much, and few of my contemporaries would claim that our generation of medical students was
abstemious.

But our drunkenness was on a different scale. In the late 1940s
we could afford to get drunk on maybe two nights a week. Now
many young people can afford to get drunk nearly every night.

Acceptable drug; unacceptable addicts

Our eagerness to turn a blind eye to the effects of alcohol
drinking on not just the young but the middle-aged members of
the business community derives from a reluctance to think of
alcohol as a drug.

The reluctance is understandable.

Alcohol drinking is deeply interwoven into patterns of Western culture and people drink not just because they like the taste
of the beer or the wine or the whisky, or because they want to
change their mood, but because drinking is part of a multitude of
social rituals, and a common lubricant of business deals.

If we want to drink sensibly – in a way which will not interfere
with our health or with our work – we need first to look at some of
the mythology that has been created around drinking.

In the past people have taken two quite different attitudes
towards those who drink too much.

The first blames the alcohol itself for the damage it causes and
seeks to banish 'the evils of drink' by banning it or severely
restricting its use. This attitude found political expression in the
temperance movement that flourished during the late nineteenth
century and in the early part of this, and in the United States led
eventually to the introduction of Prohibition.

The social disasters that Prohibition created – the glamorisa-
tion of law-breaking and the institutionalisation of crime – led to

Here's looking at you

Every year a former patient of mine, president of a division of a multinational conglomerate, gives up alcohol for Lent – not to mortify the flesh but to prove to himself that he can go for six weeks without a drink.

I suspect he's trying to exorcise a fear that haunts many of us who have a drink on most days of our lives. Though we don't drink heavily we may catch ourselves looking forward to a drink and begin to wonder whether we're becoming dependent upon it.

Our fear is fuelled by snippets of news: 'Alcohol causes death of one in four middle-aged men in Oxford Region'; 'Research into diseases caused by alcohol shows company directors are a high risk group, particularly those who travel frequently overseas.'

Once upon a time I let items like that pass me by. Every society has killjoys who revel in condemning what the rest of us enjoy. I'd looked after a dozen or so alcoholics and thought of them as people who were different from the rest of us.

Most were sad creatures but also a terrible burden on all around them: difficult to care for, untrustworthy, essentially incurable. Only a few were helped by Alcoholics Anonymous.

The relatives who sacrificed themselves to care for loved ones won my sympathy more easily than the alcoholics themselves who seemed to live in a different world from that inhabited by other people.

Then the BBC invited me to make a television series called *O'Donnell Investigates Booze* and when my friends heard the title they assumed, because I'm far from a teetotaller, that I was about to reveal the findings of a lifetime of research.

The joke wore thin when I started to investigate the drinking habits of my fellow citizens. What I found didn't put me off the stuff but it gave me a nasty shock. I discovered, not for the first time, that my attitudes were founded on experience which, while I was busy looking in other directions, time had passed by.

wider acceptance of a second attitude based on the proposition that alcohol itself is not dangerous but is abused by a minority of people who have an innate inability to handle it.

The flaw, according to this doctrine, lies not in the drink but in the drinker. Every community has a group of people different from the rest of us who, through some fault in their make-up or in their upbringing, can't 'handle' their drinking.

Countries which wanted to avoid Prohibition eagerly embraced this proposition and doctors tried to understand and treat a disease called alcoholism and patients called alcoholics.

Since the 1960s, however, scientific researchers have accrued impressive evidence that the flaw does not lie in the individual but that alcohol abuse is linked to the general availability of alcohol and to its consumption not by a genetically programmed or 'sick' minority but by us all.

Most of us don't know how great the problem is until it strikes close to home because so many people suffer the effects behind closed doors and when drunkenness erupts in the streets we call it something else, like hooliganism.

I'm not advocating prohibition. I just want to stress that those who are at special risk – and business executives are members of a high risk group – should be aware that addiction to alcohol is not something that affects a few aberrant individuals. Any of us can become addicted if we drink too much.

How can you decide whether your drinking is getting out of hand?

- my patient who gave up each Lent (see page 141) had found a convenient way to test himself. If you can go for a long spell without drinking, you are not addicted.

- another way is to keep a diary for a week just to see how much you really are consuming as opposed to what you think you are. For many people the very act of keeping the diary cuts the amount they drink.

What sort of limits should you set yourself?

For too long, doctors have offered wishy-washy advice like 'Cut down on your drinking' or 'Moderate drinking will do you no harm' without answering the $64,000 question: What is moderate drinking?

Now that researchers have redirected their attention from 'alcoholics' to the problems that can affect us all, they have got the data to define levels of alcohol intake which will not damage the liver or any other organ in the body, and which are unlikely to cause addiction.

> Recommended limits

Drinking levels are measured in units: one unit is a half pint of beer, or a standard single shot of spirits, or a glass of wine.

- if you regularly consume more than 28 units a week – 20 units for women, who are more susceptible to the effects of alcohol – you need to cut back.

- if you drink more than 35 units a week – 25 for women – you are in danger of doing yourself physical damage and run a very real risk of becoming addicted. If your drinking is at that level, it's certainly time you sought medical advice. You may not have yet damaged your health but you need to know.

A healthy attitude to drinking

Alcohol gives pleasure to millions of people who associate drinking with celebration, with relaxing with friends, with escaping from drudgery.

Alcohol, when abused, becomes associated with illness and unremitting misery for millions of 'problem drinkers' and their families.

I would suggest that a sane, and therefore healthy, attitude towards alcohol is to accept the pleasures of moderate drinking, which is now a definable entity, and to recognise the dangers of immoderate drinking.

Those of us who are at special risk should monitor our own

drinking and seek help if we find we constantly stray beyond the defined limits.

We should also as citizens be prepared to pay more for our pleasure because it is clear that raising the price of drink reduces the amount of 'problem drinking' and the number of 'problem drinkers'.

We must also recognise that these 'problem drinkers' are not a special group of diseased and inadequate people – though they may well become highly troublesome people when their addiction has taken hold – but are people like us, who didn't keep their drinking within the limits and are having to suffer the consequences.

Cutting back on unwanted drinks

Alcohol is such a common lubricant of business transactions that it's often difficult to cut back on your drinking, especially when you're in the presence of heavy drinkers who, after they've had a few drinks, are easily antagonised by anyone who refuses to keep up with them. What can you do?

- the best way to cope with the problem is not to drink at all. 'I've given it up for Lent' may be an acceptable excuse in some circles. A more effective one is to claim your doctor has put you off the booze because of a liver infection. Most people now accept this as a reasonable excuse – a liver infection is not seen as a physical defect, more an Act of God – and it has the additional advantage that, far from breeding antagonism, it can actually generate sympathy.

  If you use this ploy you will also discover the advantages that accrue to a person who really has got a clear head when dealing with those who only think their heads are clear.

- having to drive is now an acceptable excuse in all but the most hardened circles. If it doesn't work, don't be tempted to use the car anyway. Apart from the risk to life and limb, the cost of an occasional taxi is much less than the hire of a car for the year or more you could be banned.

- most of us tend to drink what we have in our hand, so when lunching or dining make sure you have a glass of water to hand as well as wine. It doesn't have to be fancy mineral water. A jug of old fashioned tap water on the table may help you cut your alcohol consumption by half.

- in a pub or at a bar try drinking wine mixed half and half with mineral water or soda. Your palate may object – it could do anyway at the wines sold by the glass in most bars – but your brain won't.

- when it's your round you can buy yourself a single instead of a double, or a drink that only looks like your previous one. Ginger ale looks like Scotch and ginger ale: straight tonic looks like gin and tonic, especially with added ice and lemon.

- better still, be honest about your look-alikes. Drinks manufacturers have responded to the consumer demand for safe drinks by producing alcohol-free beers and wines.

Cross your Heart and Hope to Live

A twentieth century plague

The publicity has blazed so fiercely there surely can be few folk left who don't know that a plague of heart disease now affects the Western world. In the world of business it is the commonest disease to afflict middle-aged men at the peak of their powers.

Impressive skills have been marshalled to deal with it. The past thirty years have seen enormous advances in the diagnosis and treatment of heart disease: coronary care units, open heart surgery, effective new drugs, implanted pacemakers, hundreds of sophisticated technical advances.

But the plague continues, claiming 180,000 victims a year in Britain – one every four minutes.

The World Health Organisation has sifted the evidence and promulgated advice on how we could lower our risk of the disease dramatically by:

- not smoking cigarettes
- having our blood pressures checked and controlled
- keeping the fat content of our diet down to 30 per cent or less of our calorie intake
- not becoming overweight
- taking regular exercise which makes our hearts beat faster

Anyone who reads newspapers and magazines will have read the advice a hundred times and, in 1987, the British government launched a £2.5 million campaign to tell people the changes they

Mangled information about risk

The decisions we need to make to protect ourselves against heart disease are not difficult to define but, because they involve people having to climb out of some comfortable ruts, they get curiously mangled in the public consciousness.

In 1987, when researching a television programme, I went to a shopping precinct in Staines in Middlesex to ask people about their attitude to the official advice they were getting on how to avoid heart disease.

Roughly a third seemed well informed and had acted on the advice. A third were well informed but had not acted. The attitude of the remaining third is summed up in this brief selection from their comments.

'My dad smoked sixty a day till he was ninety and never had a day's illness in his life.'

'Doctors are all the same. If you enjoy anything, they tell you it's bad for your health.'

'I think you can create heart disease through listening too much to what they say. Don't eat this, don't eat that, and all this nonsense.'

'How come I knew a man who didn't smoke, went jogging every day, was careful about his weight, and one day suddenly dropped dead of a heart attack?'

'Why bother? We all have to die of something, don't we?'

One cause of this mangling of information is that the doctors who give the advice seriously underrate the problem some people have in understanding concepts used in medicine, particularly the concepts of 'death rates' and 'risk factors'.

A lot of people react with the simple logic of the town clerk in a small town in the Midwest of the United States who, when the National Census Board asked for the local death rate replied quite logically: 'Same as usual. Just one per person.'

need to make in their lives to lower their risk of heart disease. We now wait to see if official exhortations will be translated into personal decisions.

Are you in the running for a heart attack?

Doctors face a problem when they talk about the 'risk factors' linked with coronary heart disease because many people find it difficult to grasp the notion of risk (see page 147) as it applies to health.

Yet, in one area of our national life, we British are obsessed with risk factors. We just call them something else.

Some of our most venerated national institutions are race-courses and, when I did some recent research at Kempton Park, I found the punters as dedicated as ever to the rigorous and hard-nosed assessment of risk factors.

They were under no illusion that they were dealing with certainty and, to help them measure risk, they used textbooks crammed with statistical and genetic information. They called them form books. They also had expert advisers whose recommendations were printed on the back pages of newspapers, and most of the punters claimed that, after much painful and expensive experience, they had become better than average at predicting results.

Their activities illustrated perfectly why the notion of risk factors is not a mathematical but a biological entity. True the assessment is based on data – the genetic and statistical information in the form books – and a mathematician who felt so inclined might consider extending the statistical data in less obvious ways.

He might, for instance, study the detailed anatomy of the horses – measuring size of muscle, length of bone, joint mobility, angle of insertion of muscles, and try to work out each animal's mechanical efficiency – but because racing punters, like doctors, are dealing not with physics but with biology, the theoretical mathematical assessment would not necessarily be a reliable indicator of performance. As many a 'good judge of horseflesh' will be happy to testify.

In biology there is often such a complex interaction of different factors, some of them maybe unknown to us, that what doctors calculate is not outcome but risk. So do the punters at Kempton Park who present their assessment of risk in a mathematical form they call odds.

I suspect that if doctors, instead of talking about risk factors, started to quote odds, people would find it easier to understand what they meant. And indeed, a few years ago, the BBC persuaded Professor Geoffrey Rose, then a member of the World Health Organisation (WHO) working party on coronary heart disease to play the part of a bookie and, using published data, quote us some odds in the Coronary Stakes.

When I went to Kempton Park, I had little trouble picking out some likely runners: not on the course but in the crowd. If the crowd was anywhere near a cross-section of the British public, I knew that one in three of the men would one day die of a heart attack as would one in four of the women.

Yet I also knew, as punters, they would be less interested in the general risk than in the risk they each ran as an individual. So I looked at the odds a bookie would lay against some of them in a race to have a coronary within the next fifteen years.

My first runner was a man, in his early thirties, who was smoking. Cigarette smokers are the favourites in this race and my WHO bookie offered odds of 9/2.

My next runner was another smoker. He has the same odds as the first save that, if the medical form book revealed that he also had raised blood pressure, his odds would shorten from 9/2 to 11/4.

Though dominated by men, the race is not restricted to them. A runner who crops up often in the form book is a woman in her thirties, on the Pill, and with raised blood pressure. Her odds would be 13/1. But if she also smoked, her odds would shorten dramatically to 5/2.

A man whose diet was high on animal fat would come under starter's orders at round about 15/2. If he were also overweight, took little exercise, and smoked, he would become the clear favourite and you'd be lucky to get odds of 9/4.

We mustn't forget the outsiders because that's what we all want to be. A man with none of the risk factors has only a 15/1 chance of having a coronary before he reaches the age of sixty and a woman with no risk factors is a rank outsider at 50/1. When we compare these outsiders with the favourites, the risk each runs becomes all too clear:

THE CORONARY STAKES	
Man on diet high in animal fat, overweight, and smoker	9/4
Woman on Pill, raised blood pressure and smoker	5/2
Man who smokes cigarettes and has raised blood pressure	11/4
Man who smokes cigarettes	9/2
Woman on Pill who has raised blood pressure	13/1
Man on diet high in animal fat	15/2
Man with no risk factors	15/1
Woman with no risk factors	50/1

As every punter knows, that list is an expression not of certainty but of likelihood – an astute and well-informed bookie's assessment of risk.

If you want to lower your risk of a coronary, first place yourself in our list of declared runners.

Then, because this is a race which nobody wants to win, if you find yourself up among the favourites, you must set about lengthening your odds:

Our favourite is a man who is overweight, eats a lot of animal fat, and smokes cigarettes
Yet if our favourite were to give up smoking he would drop dramatically down the field to the 15/2 mark. And he'd drop back pretty quickly. Within a year of stopping smoking, he'd have halved his risk and, after five years or more, his risk would be the same as that of someone who'd never smoked.

The effect on our woman smoker is even more dramatic. If she gave up smoking, she would end eventually right at the back of the field alongside our other 50/1 outsider.

Smoking is one of the main causes of heart disease. Indeed it leads to more deaths from heart attack than from any other disease, including lung cancer and chronic bronchitis. The increased risk is particularly high in smokers under fifty whose death rate from heart attack is up to ten times greater than that of non-smokers of the same age.

Once our favourite has given up smoking, he could lengthen

his odds even further if he were to alter his diet and lose some weight. Indeed he could drop as far down the field as a man can get. He has two good reasons for altering the balance of his diet:

- people who become substantially overweight before middle age, and who stay overweight, are shortening their odds dangerously and unnecessarily.

- most people in Britain eat more fat than their bodies need and a high level of animal fat in our blood – the fat that comes from fat meat and dairy products – can lead to changes in our arteries which lead eventually to a heart attack. These days many doctors will do a routine check on the cholesterol content of your blood – a measure of the fat content – and may suggest treatment to lower it.

Even a man who is not overweight can move himself to the back of the field if he reduces the fat in his diet. The sort of foods to eat are those spelled out in *Sense and nonsense about diet* (pages 105–23). Eating the right foods is no great penance. The whole point of healthy eating is that you should enjoy it.

If our favourite demotes himself, our new front runner is a woman. What can she do to lengthen her odds?
The woman who started at number two on the board would drop back to the 9/2 mark if she weren't on the Pill. And if she were also to give up smoking she would drift right to the back of the field and end up alongside the other outsiders.

Oral contraceptives are generally safe for young women to use but a woman who is over thirty-five and a smoker should consider using other methods of contraception and consult a doctor about the advisability of having short breaks during which she gives up the Pill.

The leader then would be the smoker with raised blood pressure. What can he do about that?
He most likely knows he has raised blood pressure because his doctor has told him. It's not as frightening as it sounds. In the Western world one person in five has raised blood pressure and these days doctors can do something about it. This chap may be

given tablets (see next section) which will lower his blood pressure and will also lower his odds. But there's something much more effective he can do to help himself.

Cigarettes are a far greater threat to his health than his blood pressure. And if he were to give up smoking he could move himself to the back of the field.

Our other runner with blood pressure, a woman, will also, once it's under control, move to the back of the field.

That leaves us with one clear favourite in this race to the death And of course he's a smoker. If we could only get him to give up, we'd have a race in which there would be no favourites – only outsiders.

Swinging the odds in your favour

If you want to lengthen the odds on your having a heart attack the guidelines are simple:

- **Most important of all, don't smoke**
  Smoking dramatically increases the risk of heart attacks, especially in young people

- **Eat less animal fat**
  Especially important for people who have a raised blood cholesterol level. But all of us need to reduce the amount of animal fat in our diet

- **Watch your weight**
  Particularly in early and middle life

- **Take regular exercise**
  It doesn't have to be all that vigorous. Just enough to make you a little breathless, work up a sweat, and make your heart beat faster. Swimming is fine or just brisk walking. Thirty to forty-five minutes exercise each week has been shown to halve the risk of heart attack in middle-aged people

- **Get your doctor to check your blood pressure**
  If it's raised, it can be lowered

Can you succeed in business without having a heart attack?

Business executives had a nasty shock in the early 1970s when word got round that people whose personalities led them to indulge in what was called Type A behaviour ran double the normal risk of heart disease.

Type A persons had a compelling urge to get things done in a hurry, were deeply involved in their jobs, and were aggressive competitors. To many managers, the symptoms read more like a recipe for success than a recipe for ill health. Their choice seemed to lie between having a heart attack or being a business failure.

Though later studies suggested the risk was not as great as was first feared, echoes of the original scare linger on.

More recent research suggests that Type A behaviour was too broad a definition and the only component of it linked with heart disease is one less likely to terrify managers.

There's now persuasive evidence that the component which predisposes to heart disease is a form of angry hostility which grows from Type A man's cynical lack of trust towards others, a belief that he can't depend on people being nice to him, a conviction that most people are going to be mean to him.

An American professor of psychiatry, Dr Redford B. Williams, narrows the definition even further. He says the real culprit is not the hostile anger itself but its suppression. The personality at risk is one which directs the anger inwards rather than releasing it in a dramatic outburst.

Business executives should find this refinement reassuring because it no longer indicts their sense of urgency or their sense of involvement in their jobs. The personality trait Professor Williams describes does exist in business but is nowhere near as common as the broader Type A.

Advice for those who find themselves in hostile conflict with their working environment can be found on pages 15–23.

A good way to keep up to date on how to cut your risk of heart disease is to read the first rate newsletter produced by the British Heart Foundation. The foundation, a charity based at 102 Gloucester Place, London W1H 4DH (tel: 01-935 0185), also produces authoritative and clearly written leaflets on all aspects of heart disease.

The ways of cutting the risk are easy to define, even if they are occasionally fudged by those who have a vested interest in preserving the status quo – a group which includes not just the tobacco companies but individuals who would rather rationalise their behaviour than change it.

Yet in Britain this simple advice on risk is more often offered than acted upon.

The sad truth is that if an international version of the Coronary Stakes were to be run, Britain would come romping home first. Our incidence of coronary heart disease remains the highest in the world. Hardly something to be proud of when we are talking about a literal race to the death . . . and for most of the victims a premature death.

Hypertension: how to enjoy high pressure living

'You doctors must deal with a lot of stress illness,' said a journalist friend. 'Every second article in your journals seems to be about hypertension.'

In one way he was wrong. Hypertension does not, as many people think, mean 'overtense'. It just means raised blood pressure.

In another way he was right. Hypertension *is* one of the commonest conditions that doctors see. One in five of you who read this page probably has it though many of you won't know because it doesn't make you feel ill and rarely causes symptoms.

People usually learn they have raised blood pressure when they go for an insurance medical or visit their doctor about something else. Many doctors now do a routine blood pressure check because, though they don't know the cause of most cases of

hypertension, they know enough about its management to reduce the risks it poses.

You shouldn't be afraid of having that routine check – some
department stores have installed machines on which you can
check your own pressure – because raised blood pressure doesn't
turn you into an invalid. You can still go on playing squash or
golf. You don't have to give up walking or gardening or any other
exercise you enjoy. Indeed, your doctor may encourage you to
take more exercise.

Most people with hypertension live healthy, energetic lives.
Their blood pressure causes no symptoms; they don't even feel
ill. So why should they bother to do anything about it?

There's a straightforward reason.

Though blood pressure that is raised for a short time does little
harm, pressure that remains raised for years can increase the risk
of a heart attack, a stroke, or of kidney disease. Once you know
your pressure is raised, you can do something to bring it down
and immediately reduce that risk.

Only in about five out of every hundred people with hypertension can doctors identify a specific cause: kidney disease,
glandular problems or, in women, pregnancy or the Pill. In the
remaining ninety-five, we don't know the cause, though we have
suspicions and some clues.

There's evidence, for instance, that a tendency towards raised
blood pressure can be inherited, that it may be aggravated by
constant stress, that it can be related to being overweight.
There's also evidence that relates it to a disturbance of the
mechanism by which our bodies handle the salt we consume.

One thing which makes tracking down a cause difficult is the
wide range of blood pressure found in healthy people. Like
height or weight, blood pressure is the product of myriad influences and some people's blood pressure may be 'raised' only
because they are at the extreme end of the normal range. The
range of pressure found in healthy people means you really need
to consult a doctor to discover whether your pressure at your age
is at a level you should do something about.

Positive action

Your first reaction to hearing your blood pressure is raised may be that you're now an invalid and your days of normal living are over. Not true.

Nor are you likely to have a stroke at any minute. Indeed, the advantage of discovering your blood pressure is raised is that you can *reduce* your risk of having a stroke.

Nor are you going to have to live a mollycoddled life and give up many of the things you enjoy.

'Doing something about' your blood pressure will probably involve making adjustments to your style of living. But you'll be happy to discover there are many more 'Dos' than 'Don'ts'.

- **Do exercise**
  A doctor who finds your blood pressure raised will probably advise you to take some healthy exercise every day. That doesn't mean jogging or 'physical jerks'. Healthy exercise is activity which makes your heart beat faster and makes you work up a mild sweat; above all, it is exercise you enjoy.

  A brisk walk you enjoy is better than a work-out which you don't, and you can take your healthy exercise swimming, cycling, playing tennis or football, or taking part in any other competitive sport. If you have the most common form of hypertension, exercise, far from harming you, will do you good, particularly if you enjoy it.

- **Don't smoke**
  This is the only real 'Don't'. Cigarettes are a much greater threat to your health than is your blood pressure and it's foolish to run that risk while you're trying to get your blood pressure under control.

- **Do watch your weight**
  If you're overweight, you'll need to lose some. For many people, as their weight begins to fall, so does their blood pressure. You don't have to go on a rigid diet, just learn how to eat more sensibly. So you can still enjoy your food while

getting the balance right: less fat, sugar, and salt, more fibre. (See page 107, *Sense and nonsense about diet*.)

Remember that sugar that's been refined – separated from its fibre – can supply the energy you need, but that's all it does supply. Unrefined sugar – found in fruit, vegetables, cereals, and pulses – supplies not just energy but fibre. Eaten this way it's more filling and makes it less easy for you to take the excess calories that could make you overweight. It's easier to swallow those extra, fattening, calories in the refined sugar added to confectionery, sauces, and many canned goods.

- **Do cut down on animal fat**
Our main source of animal fat is not fatty meat but dairy products. But eating less fat doesn't mean eating no dairy products.

Try semi-skimmed milk instead of gold or silver top; you'll find it hard to tell the difference. Even better, try skimmed milk; you may detect a difference but you may not mind it. To cut down on butter, try low fat spreads or margarine. And don't forget: cakes and biscuits contain lots of hidden fat.

Another worthwhile change is to replace some of the animal fat in your diet with the polyunsaturated fats which are found in sunflower, safflower, maize, fish oils, and some margarines. Food cooked in oil is certainly healthier, and usually more enjoyable, than food fried in fat. (See also pages 105–23.)

- **Do cut down on salt**
The part salt plays in raising blood pressure is not completely clear. As yet there's no convincing evidence that if we all took less salt, fewer of us would get hypertension. But there is evidence that people who have raised blood pressure can reduce it slightly if they cut their salt intake. (See page 113.) A low salt diet also increases the efficiency of some blood pressure-lowering drugs.

So, if you have hypertension, it would seem sensible to take less salt. There's no need to use salt substitutes – they could do you more harm than good. Just don't put salt on the table, use too much in cooking, or eat heavily salted foods.

- **Do eat more fibre**
  This is easy. You just have to eat more fresh fruit and vegetables, including potatoes, and more salads, nuts, wholemeal bread and cereals, beans and other pulses.

- **Do watch how much alcohol you drink**
  If you're a heavy drinker, you should aim to become a 'moderate' drinker. You don't have to go on the wagon, unless you want to. Indeed some doctors think 'moderate drinking' can help you, though their evidence is less strong than it once appeared.
  The $64,000 question is what is 'moderate drinking' It's easier to say what is dangerous drinking. Drinking levels are measured in units (see page 143, *The Trouble with Booze*). There's one unit in half a pint of beer, a single shot of spirits, or a glass of wine. A man who consumes more than 28 units a week needs to cut back. Women are more susceptible to the effects of alcohol and the upper limit for them is 20 units.

- **Do learn to relax**
  Doctors still argue over the part that stress plays in raising blood pressure, other than for a short time, but there's no denying that a lot of people can lower their pressure with relaxation techniques which range from simple muscle relaxation exercises and self-hypnosis to transcendental meditation. If I had hypertension, I would certainly try to learn those techniques.

Drugs

A major advance in medicine over the past twenty years has been the development of drugs which lower raised blood pressure and so cut the risk associated with hypertension. These drugs fall into different groups, each lowering blood pressure in a different way.

- **Beta-blockers**
  Act on the nerves that control the circulation in a way that reduces blood pressure

- **Diuretics**
  Produce the same effect by causing the kidneys to excrete more salt and water

- **Vasodilators**
  Widen the diameter of the small arteries in the body, so reducing the resistance to the flow of blood and the pressure needed to drive it through

- **Calcium antagonists**
  Produce the same sort of effect as vasodilators

- **ACE inhibitors**
  Antagonise a hormone which raises blood pressure

These are the main groups but there are others, and you really need expert medical advice on which is the right drug for you. The choice is affected by the sort of hypertension you have, the level to which your pressure is raised, and your individual medical history.

The choice is also affected by unwanted effects of the drugs in some individuals. A particular beta-blocker may cause excessive lassitude in one person but not in another. If you need to take tablets to lower your blood pressure your doctor may in the early stages have to keep varying the drug, and the dose, until he finds the combination that is right for you.

Not everybody with hypertension needs a drug but those who do have to accept what seems a bizarre routine: taking tablets every day though they feel perfectly well, to treat something which has never caused them problems, probably never will, and which they didn't know they had until it was discovered by chance. Small wonder that many give up the tablets or forget to take them. Yet, if they do, and their blood pressure goes up again, they are back in their previous state of risk.

Far from being a death sentence, discovering your blood pressure is raised can actually improve your enjoyment of life. Many businessmen and women find that adjusting their style of living opens up new areas of interest and fulfilment.

What a lot of executives enjoy most is the cast iron excuse they have for dropping activities which were beginning to bore them and which they were continuing largely out of habit. It's more than adequate compensation for having to take those tablets.

How to Avoid Cancer

Cancer can be avoided. Cancer can be prevented. Cancer can be cured.

If you want to learn why those three statements will come as a surprise to most people in Britain, and will be disbelieved by many, then read on.

If you're in a hurry to find out how to protect yourself, turn now to 'Positive action' (page 171) which offers seven practical guidelines for avoiding cancer. The earlier sections deal with the reasoning and evidence that underpin those guidelines.

The disease that dare not speak its name

When my favourite uncle was not busy being my uncle he was the secretary of the Ford Motor Company in Ireland. One talent which had earned him his success in business was his lively intelligence, yet when he developed cancer twenty years ago every member of his family was ordered not to tell him the nature of his illness.

According to my aunt, even the Dublin surgeon who made the diagnosis couldn't bring himself to name the disease.

Hesitantly she asked: 'Tell me doctor, is it . . . ?'

But, before she could complete the sentence, the surgeon replied: 'Yes it is. I'm afraid it's the Big Fellah.'

Twenty years later most of us seem no braver at naming names. In 1984 I made a television series called *How to Avoid Cancer* and before we started, the BBC's Broadcasting Research Department asked a thousand people, a 'nationally representative sample', about their attitudes to cancer and followed up the interviews with a series of group discussions.

To most of the interviewees, cancer was frightening, alien, fatal, incurable, taboo-ridden, and mysterious. They thought it had no obvious causes and could not be prevented. Their emotional reaction was one of dread and superstition.

Little comfort there for doctors who think they've made a reasonable job of keeping their patients well informed. But then doctors themselves are not immune to superstition.

While I was making that television series and people asked me what I was working on, not once did I hear myself give the straight reply. Instead I heard decorated answers – 'A series on cancer. I get all the cheerful subjects.' As if I needed to add a protective prayer after speaking the forbidden word.

Cancer mythology

The BBC research revealed that the irrational fears and ideas people have about cancer derive from one central misunderstanding. Most of those interviewed saw cancer as a single disease which 'breaks out' in different parts of the body rather than as what it is: a group of diseases with only one mechanism in common – body cells breaking the rules of growth.

Few interviewees understood that cancers have different causes, run different courses, and respond differently to different forms of treatment.

But then most people talk of cancer in the singular – cancers would be more accurate – and the notion that this single disease lurks within a person, maybe from birth, until it chooses its moment to strike, or is provoked by a knock or a shock, gives it the mystique of a medieval curse visited upon unfortunates.

Said one interviewee: 'Often people don't like to say someone is suffering from it. Or if you speak to somebody and they've got it they don't want to tell you. Almost like leprosy.'

The BBC survey also revealed that, maybe out of dread, people don't try to seek out the 'hard facts' about cancer in the way they do with heart disease or other serious illnesses. Their information consists of snippets – some true, some false – that they have picked up from long-forgotten sources and have never tried to organise into an understandable whole. These collections of snippets lead to bizarre misunderstandings. Some information has got through but it's been curiously mangled in transmission.

Nearly 90 per cent of interviewees, for instance, nominated smoking as a cause of cancer. Yet many challenged their own opinion with their experience. Because they thought smoking was an inevitable 'cause' of cancer – which it is not, though it greatly increases the risk – smokers who didn't get lung cancer were adduced as evidence against any link:

'My uncle and aunt smoked until they were nearly 90 and they just died of old age.'

And many thought smoking was linked to *all* cancers. So again their experience subverted their opinion:

'My Mum and Dad both died of it – theirs was in their tummy – and yet they say that smoking causes cancer and neither of those two smoked.'

This confusion over possible causes leads to the 'nothing and everything' attitude of the saloon bar philosopher. One minute he will say: 'Nothing actually *causes* your cancer. I mean there's no direct link, no *cause and effect* that your experts have actually *proved*.'

Yet, five minutes later he will announce with equal vehemence: 'These days *everything* causes cancer. Coffee, drink, fags, sex. I mean, what's left for a man to do? You name it; they tell you not to do it.'

The attitude is easy to understand. Professor Sir Richard Doll, former professor of medicine at Oxford and an international authority on cancer epidemiology, has pointed out that so many things *may* cause cancer you're a lucky person if you get out of this world alive. And when so many things seem to be indicted people feel it's not really worth trying to give anything up.

The trouble with the nothing and everything syndrome is that, while many causes are named, even accepted in a half-hearted way, none is actually believed – believed to the extent that people will act on the belief.

No one, for instance, has shown that cigarette smoking *causes* lung cancer but many have shown that stopping smoking will dramatically reduce an individual's risk of getting the disease.

Once people realise that they can tilt the odds in their favour without having to wait for absolute proof of a *cause*, they are more likely to take action to protect themselves.

The tragedy of the misunderstanding that now prevails, and of the superstition it generates, is that many cancers that could be prevented are not being prevented.

Tragedy is not an overstatement. Our reluctance to talk about the disease means that few people know that about 40 per cent – yes, 40 per cent – of cancer deaths in Britain are preventable, that nearly 59,000 people in the UK die unnecessarily of cancer every year.

And prevention is not difficult.

Organising your defences

Smoking

We could prevent a third of those unnecessary deaths, at a proverbial stroke, if people stopped smoking cigarettes. Lung cancer is the commonest lethal cancer in the United Kingdom. Repetition of the warning – and propaganda from the tobacco industry – seems to have dulled our sensitivity to what are horrifying figures.

One in every four smokers will be killed before their time by their addiction and, in Britain, cigarette smoking now kills *four* times as many people as are killed by drink, drugs, murder, suicide, road, rail or air accidents, poisoning, drowning, fires, falls, and every other known cause of accidental death, all lumped together.

The good news is that it's never too late to stop smoking cigarettes. Your risk of lung cancer starts to diminish from the day you give up, no matter how long you've been a smoker. Equally good news is that increasingly sophisticated help is at hand.

If you have a problem stopping smoking, your doctor can help you by suggesting devices – the most popular is a chewing gum –

that will supply you with a graduated dose of nicotine to insulate you against the sudden withdrawal of that drug. Your local health centre can also put you in touch with self-help groups where ex-smokers and others trying to break the habit give one another moral support and swap practical tips based on their own experience.

As it happens, most people still kick the addiction by sheer determination. Many reinforce their determination by planning to stop on a certain day and telling everyone around them of their intention, so that any backsliding will mean a loss of face. Stopping smoking is clearly the most effective step anyone can take to avoid cancer.

But there are others.

A growing number of nutritional scientists and cancer specialists now believes that what we eat may turn out to be as significant as what we smoke.

Diet

Sir Richard Doll suggests that maybe a third of all cancers are caused by elements in our diet which we could easily modify. He admits he's not stating an absolute percentage that he can prove, but claims it is a reasonable estimate based on some evidence and some guesswork by people with wide experience in cancer research. If their guesswork is wildly wrong, the figure might be as low as 10 per cent but Sir Richard wouldn't be surprised if it turned out to be a good deal higher – 50 or even 70 per cent.

Most cancers take a long time to develop. So when we look for foods that may have caused the cancers people are getting now, we're not looking for new foods, or for recent additives to food, but for foods they've been eating for some time.

There's little evidence, for instance, to support the popular notion that the chemicals added during modern food processing cause cancer. These have to pass stringent tests before manufacturers can add them to food and, far from being a danger, they can help protect us by preserving the food from the sort of deterioration that produces cancer-causing chemicals.

Some years ago there was a scare when research – largely

prompted by the sugar industry – showed that artificial sweeteners (cyclamates and saccharin) could cause cancer in animals. But the amounts involved were equivalent to human beings adding 7 or 8 lbs of the stuff to a cup of tea. Scientists now think that the risk from sweeteners, if it exists at all, is likely to be very small.

The most exciting information we have about diet is not about additives and chemicals but about the way the nature of the whole diet can affect a person's risk of getting certain cancers. This knowledge came first from a study of the differing pattern of cancers in different countries.

The differences are unmistakable. Breast cancer and colon cancer are major killers in the affluent countries of the West but are rare in poorer developing countries. Japan has high rates of stomach cancer but low rates of breast and colon cancer.

These differences in cancer patterns seem to be linked to differences in diet. The Japanese who get stomach cancer, for instance, are those who eat a lot of highly spiced, salted, and pickled food.

As yet we do not have hard scientific proof that differences in diet *cause* certain cancers but they do seem to affect the *risk*. That means that, by altering our diet, we can tilt the odds in our favour.

Some of the most impressive evidence on diet comes from studies of emigrant populations. Africans and Japanese who emigrate to the USA eventually get cancers that are rare in their native countries and common in their host country. Even Japanese living in Japan are now beginning to get a Western pattern of cancers as they adopt an increasingly Westernised diet.

Neither the Eastern nor the Western diet is ideal but scientists are beginning to track down the elements in each that increase – or decrease – the risk of cancer. And they now know enough about those elements to recommend changes in eating habits that would help us all to avoid cancer.

They have a lot of evidence which suggests that increasing the fibre in our diet – eating wholemeal bread instead of white, eating more potatoes, more cereals and pulses – reduces our risk of

Cancer and lifestyle in North America

The Mormons who live in Utah suffer about one third the number of cancers suffered by non-Mormons living in the same state. Their style of living – now much studied by scientists – differs from that of most other US citizens. Fewer Mormons smoke and their diet is very different from the usual US diet:

- they grow their own food, mill their grain, and eat more of it
- they eat more cereals, fruit, and vegetables
- they eat less meat, and drink less coffee and tea
- many fewer of them drink alcohol

Because we're talking about risks and not causes, no one can guarantee you won't get cancer if you adopt that style of life. But you will reduce your risk.

And, if you add some daily exercise, you'll also protect yourself against heart disease.

getting cancer, particularly cancers of the bowel and breast. And they have evidence that we can reduce our risk by eating more green vegetables and more fresh fruit.

They also are accumulating evidence that eating too much fat increases the risk of some cancers. Indeed many nutritional experts would like us to cut the amount of fat in our national diet by about a quarter.

Your risk of getting cancer is affected not just by the quality of your diet. Quantity can also play a part. Obesity seems to be linked to about 2 per cent of UK cancer deaths.

Alcohol

The good news for drinkers is that the risk of alcohol causing cancer is almost negligible if you don't smoke. If you do smoke –

cigarettes, pipe or cigars – then it does seem a good idea to go easy on the booze. Alcohol and tobacco smoke seem to work in combination in producing cancers of the mouth or throat, which account for about 3 per cent of cancer deaths in Britain.

To reduce that risk you need to cut your drinking to no more than three or four glasses of wine or spirits – or (larger) glasses of beer – a day.

The nice thing about the cancer experts' advice on diet and alcohol is that it is acceptable even to self-indulgent folk like me. My happiest discovery when I looked at the sort of diet they were recommending was that the foods that seem to protect us against cancer are more enjoyable to eat than those that increase our risk.

Facing up to it

Fears about cancer, based on misunderstanding and superstition, still prevent people seeking medical advice.

One of the great medical clichés, repeated in every health guide ever written, is 'If in doubt, don't sit and worry but see a doctor.'

Sadly it is advice that is still as often ignored as followed. Yet the rate at which scientific knowledge has advanced over the past decade makes it more valuable now that it has ever been. We know that early detection of some cancers greatly increases the chance of successful treatment. We suspect the same is true of many others.

There is even one potential cancer that, if detected early enough, can be cured *before* it becomes malignant. This is a cancer that affects the entrance – the cervix – of the womb.

The method of detection is the cervical smear test in which a wooden or plastic spatula is rubbed gently and painlessly across the cervix. The cells collected on the spatula are then smeared across a glass slide and examined under a microscope through which an experienced eye can detect the changes which presage the development of cancer.

At that stage, simple medical treatment can prevent the cancer from developing. The affected area is removed by a minor surgical operation – often so minor that the woman does not have to go into hospital.

Small wonder that the specialists who know they can prevent this disease regard it as a shameful tragedy that, in Britain, some 2,000 women still die each year of cancer of the cervix. Those deaths could be prevented if all women had regular cervical smear tests: the first soon after they begin their active sexual life, a second within a year, and then one every five years up to the age of sixty-five.

In 1987 a group of London doctors devised a new test which, because it replaces the lengthy microscopic examination with a simpler chemical test, may eventually speed up the diagnostic procedure.

Early warning signs

There's nothing morbid about knowing the early warning signs of cancer and looking out for them – as long as you don't let the process become an obsession that dominates your life.

The practical reason for responding to warning signs is that, if you take your cancer to a doctor earlier, not only do you have a better chance of being cured but the sort of treatment you will need may be less radical than it would be if you waited.

What things to look for?

The main one is any persistent change in what has been normal health for you. Obvious examples are unexplained and persistent bleeding, unusual weight loss, persistent pain – particularly in places where you don't normally get pain – a persistent change in bowel habit, or any persistent lump anywhere.

If a spot or 'mole' on your skin seems to be getting bigger or if a 'mole' that you have had for years starts to enlarge or to bleed, show it to a doctor. In most cases it will prove to be a harmless blemish but, if it is a skin cancer in its early stages, it can be cured.

There are also less particular symptoms: general ill-health, a general feeling of malaise, of not feeling well, of being 'run down', or 'one degree under'.

None of these signs and symptoms mean you have cancer; all of them have much more common causes. But they are signs and symptoms you should present to a doctor for evaluation.

The warning signs are easy to detect yet, sadly, even well informed and intelligent people often ignore them for an all too human reason.

One lesson I learned early in my medical career is that people who run their businesses in coolly rational style can become confusedly irrational when making decisions about their health. Their unreason is not always the product of ignorance; it is often the product of fear, particularly fear of the unknown. Seemingly intelligent people may put off taking their symptoms to a doctor because they fear not just the diagnosis of cancer but the treatment it might involve. Fear of the diagnosis derives from the belief that it is always a death sentence.

That's just not true. The past twenty years have seen the development of treatments for cancers which were previously incurable:

- only ten years ago men with a particular form of cancer of the testicle died of it; now most are cured with a new drug treatment

- most cancers in children, and many in adults, are now curable with combinations of drugs, radiotherapy, and surgery

The pessimism that dominated the cancer wards when I was a young doctor thirty years ago has been replaced by the sort of enthusiasm and energy that businessmen and women can sniff out in a successful enterprise.

There are, of course, cancers which are incurable and from which people do die. Yet even for these, modern medicine has treatments which offer patients longer lives of high quality, and protection from pain. We all suffer from an incurable disease called mortality and cancer is now a no more painful or degrading way to achieve our destiny than any other illness.

There is another fear which causes otherwise rational people to cast a blind eye at the early warning signs – the fear of cancer treatment. That fear too is no longer justified. No form of medical treatment is exactly pleasurable but cancer treatment these days is not as unpleasant as people imagine it to be.

Modern cancer experts don't indulge in a reckless chase after survival for their patients regardless of the human cost. Of course they seek treatments which will produce more 'cures' but they also seek treatments which are less unpleasant, easier to apply, quicker to act.

Positive action

We are lucky that all the cancers in which the results of treatment are disappointing are ones we should be able to prevent because they are related to our habits, to the way we live.

We are even luckier that the preventive steps we can take as individuals are simple to define and can be reduced to seven uncomplicated guidelines:

- don't smoke. And don't work in closed environments with others smoking around you. This is by far the most significant step anyone can take to cut their risk of developing a cancer. Smoking accounts for over 30 per cent of all serious cancers.

- if you *do* smoke, go easy on the alcohol. (See page 139, *The Trouble with Booze*).

- avoid obesity, which probably contributes to 2 per cent of UK cancer deaths. In women, it certainly increases the risk of cancer of the womb and is suspected to increase the risk of other cancers in men and women. Keeping your weight within decent limits will also reduce your risk of heart disease. (See page 152, *Swinging the odds in your favour*).

- all women should have a regular cervical smear test at the intervals recommended on page 169. 2,000 women still die each year of cancer of the cervix.

- take care in the sun. Overexposure to sunlight can cause skin cancers. This is a greater hazard in countries like Australia than in our cloudier northern climes but the risk does exist. Overdoing sunbathing whether it be on a beach, on a sunbed, or in a solarium will increase your risk of getting skin cancer, particularly if you have fair skin or red hair.

But don't let that increased risk drive you paranoiac. Skin cancer accounts for less than 1 per cent of all serious cancers in the UK.

- balance your diet in the way suggested in *Sense and Nonsense about Diet* (pages 105–23). Sir Richard Doll suggests that maybe a third of all cancers are diet-related. Limit the fat you eat and eat plenty of fibre and fresh fruit and vegetables.

- if your work brings you into contact with radiation, hazardous fumes or chemicals, or asbestos dust, obey the safety regulations exactly as they are stated and take no 'short cuts'. Chemicals and other substances used in industry cause about 4 per cent of serious cancers.

Following these simple guidelines won't guarantee you immunity against cancer but will greatly reduce your risk of getting it.

A Business-like Approach to Medical Treatment

When is a drug not a drug?

Potions, philtres, and medicines

I find it odd that some people who have built successful careers by taking well-informed, logical decisions in business allow one corner of their lives to be dominated by misapprehension and superstition – the corner which harbours their attitudes to medicines, as opposed to other forms of treatment.

I find it less odd when I remind myself that only in the past fifty years has science imported scepticism into a domain which for so long was the preserve of hucksters and magicians.

After centuries of love philtres and magic potions, we haven't really had time to grow used to the idea of medicines. And our understanding of them isn't helped by the fact that, despite the science, faith is still the main active ingredient in many of them.

It's easy to forget just how quickly medicines have changed. Only forty years ago when someone had a headache they didn't just reach into pocket, handbag, or bathroom cabinet in search of a proprietary remedy; they were as likely to call at their local chemist and ask him to make up a 'headache draught'.

The word 'draught' retained a link with 'potion' and many people want a similar echo of the magic past when they take a modern drug. The distinction between 'drug' and 'medicine' is purely semantic yet people are usually happier if their remedy is called a medicine rather than a drug. Drugs are nasty, dangerous things, likely to cause addiction.

Come to think of it, a lot of folk are not too happy about taking drugs even when they are called medicines. Most people are prepared to accept far greater risks with surgery than they are with 'medication', even when the objective is the elimination of the same painful or dangerous condition. (One paradoxical result of this prejudice is that doctors have accumulated much more information – and more reliable information – on the risks of 'drugs' than on the risks of other forms of treatment.)

Some of the prejudice against therapy that comes in tablet or liquid form derives from a misunderstanding. Modern drugs are seen as a development of the salves and cures of old, when potions were carefully prepared to meet specific needs: a 'nerve tonic', a potion for the gout, a potion for the liver, a 'headache draught'.

Though some manufacturers of modern drugs reinforce that misunderstanding by trading on it, today's drugs and medicines are *not* magic substances uniquely fashioned to 'cure' particular diseases; they are just chemicals which, when ingested, alter the working of our bodies in some useful ways – and also in some not so useful ways.

A drug is useful if some of the alterations it produces help the body combat the effects of a particular disease. But it is extremely rare for a drug to do only that. Most have other unwanted effects which come to be called 'side-effects'. It's an unfortunate phrase because it fosters the idea that at the centre of the drug lies a wholesome 'cure' which has been contaminated by other nasty effects which have crept into it.

The ideal medicine or drug would indeed be one which produced only the effects needed to counter a particular disease. Yet though a few drugs approach this ideal, none achieves it and treatment with medicines, like any other form of treatment – with surgery or with the new technologies – is a matter of weighing benefits against risk.

In an ideal world, all patients would, if they wanted it, be given all the information they needed to try to balance benefit against risk for themselves. Some might choose to leave the judgement to the doctor or, at least give a lot of weight to the doctor's advice, based as it is on experience and specialised knowledge.

But in the end the right to accept or reject treatment must be yours.

In the less than ideal world which most of us inhabit, you should, unless you want to delegate all responsibility, ask any doctor who offers you treatment for an explanation of all the possible effects, not just the 'good' ones.

As it happens, our thinking about medicines would be less confused if we remembered that drugs don't have intrinsically 'good' or intrinsically 'bad' effects, they just have effects, some of which help the treatment of a particular disease, some of which don't. Indeed, with drugs which are useful in treating more than one disease, the side effects in one patient may be the useful effects in another.

Mind and body

Our understanding of medicines is also clouded by non-semantic oddities, the most significant of which is the complex interplay 'twixt mind and body which occurs in every illness. (See pages 23–30.)

When new drugs are assessed in trials in which half the patients receive the drug and half an inert 'placebo', a significant proportion of patients receiving the placebo will lose their symptoms though they are having no more treatment than they were before the trial began.

This placebo effect has been the ally of hucksters down the ages and still allows people to peddle 'cures' of dubious validity. Medicines tend to work if people 'believe' in them – particularly if their doctors also 'believe' in them – and often a person's attachment to a false 'cure' causes no harm save a certain amount of pain to those who would like life to be more logical than it is.

Yet it can cause undoubted harm when it prevents people having other treatment which might be life-saving or when it encourages people who can't afford it to squander their savings on 'cures' which produce no effective improvement in the length or quality of their lives.

Sometimes the triumph of faith over logic promotes not just a 'cure' but a style of thinking based on dangerous illogicality. A good example is the current fashionable belief that there is something inherently healthy in a food or drug – or 'cure' – that is made only of natural ingredients.

Beware the 'natural' explanation

A quick tour of your friendly neighbourhood shopping centre may convince you that 'Natural' is the word on which the health food industry is founded. Yet natural foods have no intrinsic advantages over unnatural ones, indeed are often more dangerous. When I was a child I got a tuberculous gland in my neck because I drank pure natural cow's milk. If I'd had milk that had been subjected to the nasty unnatural process of pasteurisation, I would have been spared a painful operation, and my parents a great deal of worry.

In north-east Thailand, I have seen refugees suffering from cholera because they insisted on drinking water from a contaminated natural spring rather than the less attractive stuff we brought to the camps in tankers and which had been treated with unnatural chlorine.

As a doctor I don't see Nature as a benevolent matriarch. My profession spends a lot of time trying to insulate human beings from the effects of natural catastrophes or trying to repair bodies and minds that have been visited by an often malevolent Mother Nature.

Indeed medicine's job is to protect people from the ravages of our often hostile natural environment and, when protection fails, to try and repair the damage.

Naturally occurring smallpox was driven from the world by unnatural vaccination. Natural bacteria which enter our bodies and cause infections which sometimes kill are themselves destroyed by unnatural antibiotic chemicals injected through unnatural needles.

Our coroners' courts still recognise that most people die of natural causes.

But even if I weren't a doctor I would worry about the

unreason involved in nature worship because of the effect such worship has had on attitudes to progress not just in science but in enterprises which strive to improve the conditions under which we live.

I'm not suggesting we have nothing to learn from complex natural processes which have evolved through aeons of natural selection and biological adaptation.

I can understand why women are attracted to natural childbirth, though not why some are prepared to run risks with their own lives and the life of their child rather than admit that man's natural ingenuity has devised ways of averting some of the obstetrical catastrophes that nasty old Mother Nature still inflicts on childbearing women.

I'm also prepared to admit that breastfeeding is the safest, most rewarding, and least expensive way for a mother to feed a baby but I worry about the romantic and passionate – dare I call it religious – attachment to this natural process that condemns all women who are unwilling or unable – often for good medical reasons – to breastfeed their babies.

I'm aware that 'organically grown' foods command higher prices than those grown with the aid of chemical fertilisers though the scientist within me doubts whether a plant or vegetable is much concerned about the source of the molecules which it absorbs.

Belief in the 'natural goodness' of organic foods is a pretty harmless delusion but these fads grow dangerous when they are expanded to project a vision of the world in which 'nature' is Good and anything 'unnatural' is Evil. In this religion, chemical fertilisers and insecticides are immoral and technology is the work of the devil. Natural foods are the gift of the gods; drugs are dangerous man-made poisons.

That sort of unreason angers doctors of my generation. We have seen vaccines and drugs rid whole populations of infectious diseases which fifty years ago were regarded as natural pestilences. And we've seen new drugs and new technologies transform the miserable lives that had to be led by those who had the ill luck to be born with natural afflictions like asthma or gross congenital deformities.

Recently I attended a meeting convened to promote 'a natural approach to the treatment of cancer' and made myself unpopular by demanding a definition of the key word. Was it natural, I asked, for man to fly? All but one of the speakers had arrived by aeroplane. And was a cathode ray tube a natural phenomenon? All had appeared on television the night before to promote their views.

I was accused of being a 'disruptive force' and invited to remove myself. Yet, if my accusers had paused to think, they'd have realised the answer to both my questions was 'yes'. Aeroplanes and television *are* natural phenomena, invented by man who is himself part of nature and uses his natural ingenuity to protect and improve his environment.

Doctors learn early in their careers that Nature has no bias. It is neither for us nor against us. Natural laws can be defined as clearly – and work as inexorably – in the spread of an epidemic as in the birth of a healthy baby.

I see no harm in Nature being used as a generator of nostalgic packaging or of cute shop design, nor as a means of selling organically grown comestibles. I see much harm in it being used to sell untested cancer cures and quackery. And I see the greatest harm when nature worship becomes a celebration of unreason.

Medical science is merely a process of observing natural events, and, by the application of reason to our observations, trying to understand them, trying to learn from them, trying occasionally to turn them to our advantage.

Some forty years' involvement in that process has led me to conclude that man's survival on this planet depends not on worship of a non-existent Mother Nature but on dedicated employment of the natural gift of reason.

When is a risk not a risk?

Medicines are not the only substances which, when we take them into our bodies, change our internal environment. Most chemicals can, if we ingest them, alter what the French physiologist Claude Bernard called our *milieu intérieur*. And whether we call them foods, drinks, condiments, poisons, or drugs is largely a matter of historical or cultural accident.

Yet, this accidental semantic distinction influences a host of public attitudes.

Judges sipping their fourth glass of port, housewives drinking their umpteenth cup of coffee or tea, bar-side politicians chain-smoking their way through the evening think drug addiction is something that occurs in others – just as nice old souls who are happy to sprinkle salt over their potatoes will chain themselves to the waterworks railings at the mention of fluoride.

If any substance has the misfortune to be labelled a drug it is looked on in quite a different way and faces different prejudices from those it would if historical accident had labelled it a condiment or food.

Those semantic distinctions can themselves have serious side-effects.

One of Britain's most respected experts on prescription medicines believes that our confusion over the meaning of 'drug' and our ignorance of mathematics – reinforced by noisy media campaigns – have led to the premature banning of valuable drugs, including some that would have eased the lot of patients suffering from painful diseases like arthritis.

Dr Bill Inman has no ties with the pharmaceutical industry and, indeed, once worked for the government department concerned with the regulation of medicines. He is now at the University of Southampton where, as Director of the Drug Surveillance Unit, he has accumulated formidable experience in monitoring the side-effects of prescribed drugs and has often described how ignorance can lead to bizarre public attitudes towards risk.

Because ignorance breeds superstition, it shouldn't surprise us that our perception of risk owes more to primitive fear than to the mathematics of probability. And fear is more easily triggered by one major tragic event than by a series of minor ones.

Imagine what public reaction would be if four fully laden jumbo jets crashed at Heathrow Airport every week killing all passengers. Yet that is the weekly British death toll attributable to cigarettes, a toll which the British public accepts with resignation and the British government with apparent equanimity.

Our perception of risk also involves a political quality. Sir Hermann Bondi, the mathematician, has illustrated this with the tale of a Swedish plan to study the aurora borealis by firing instrument-carrying rockets into it. When the rockets had done their job, their burnt out remnants were due to fall over an area of Lapland so sparsely populated that the mathematical risk of anyone being hit was minute. Even so, the Swedish government felt it should offer protection to those who lived there. It lifted out the isolated reindeer herders by helicopter and lifted them back when the experiment was over.

Sir Hermann calculated that the mathematical likelihood of one of them being hit by a piece of rocket was less than 1 per cent of that of a helicopter accident.

He also invites us to look at the political implications. If someone had been hit – or even had had just 'a bad fright' – the Interior Minister would have faced the angry accusation that he had done nothing to protect people for whom he was responsible. On the other hand, if there had been a helicopter crash, people would have happily accepted a ministerial statement which said: 'We deeply sympathise with the relatives of the victims of this tragedy. We used a well tried helicopter, flown by a well trained and experienced crew. We are appalled at what has happened but there is no other precaution we could have taken.'

In one of his 1978 Reith Lectures, Lord Rothschild said: 'There is no point in getting into a panic about the risks of life until you have compared the risks which worry you with those that don't, but perhaps should.'

Yet Dr Inman points out that people will worry about a risk with a drug that is one thousandth of that they run every time they get into a car, that patients will happily accept a scale of risk with surgery that they would never countenance with a drug, and that only rarely does public discussion of risk include a comparative assessment of benefit.

We are right to be shocked when drug treatment causes a death but prescribed medicines come actively under suspicion when the risk of death from treatment is 100 or even 10,000 times less than the risk of death from the disease.

Indeed Dr Inman claims that Britain has banned drugs in circumstances in which the mathematical risk has never been stated, maybe never even measured.

The main thrust of his argument is that, though treatment with modern drugs is remarkably safe, we seem unable to agree what risks are acceptable in return for undeniable benefits. Public opinion, he suggests, has swung much too far in the direction of excessive concern about rare side-effects while ignoring the much more common benefits.

He calculates that if we eliminated *all* drug risks we would increase average life expectancy by thirty-seven minutes. To achieve that we would have to ban all drugs and vaccines. And that would decrease average expectancy by between ten and twenty years.

Positive action

If all of us were to apply the logic we try to bring to business decisions to decisions we have to make about our health we might develop more rational attitudes towards medical treatment.

True, the benefits of many drugs have been oversold and we are right to be sceptical of the claims of hucksters. When offered any form of treatment we should always ask what risk we are being asked to run and for what benefit.

We now know a great deal about the effects – useful and harmful – of prescription medicines and intelligent men and women should not let vaguely understood prejudices cut them off from the undoubted benefits which are available.

The prejudices affect not just major decisions about treatment but quite small ones.

I see little point, for instance, in your 'soldiering on' with a headache, or any other sort of ache, when a couple of tablets may not only ease your pain but, in doing so, improve your efficiency.

I see even less point in your taking an ineffective remedy because it is 'herbal' or 'natural' and therefore, your prejudice tells you, safer than a chemical produced in a laboratory.

It may well be much more dangerous.

How much do you want to know?

When I was a family doctor I looked after a man who had earned a reputation as a business buccaneer. He was chief executive of a large public company which he ran with the same entrepreneurial flair with which he had originally built his own private business.

Some of his fellow directors used to mutter that he ran it too much as a one-man band but the shareholders never complained or, if they felt inclined to do so, the ever increasing value of their shares and the size of their dividends were good reasons to stay silent.

My patient developed a form of cancer which, though its progress could be slowed by treatment, was destined inevitably to shorten his life. The London physician who confirmed the diagnosis wanted to fudge an explanation of the disease because he thought all patients would prefer their doctors not to hand them a death warrant.

Yet over the years I'd looked after that patient, he'd always wanted to know the exact nature of every illness he'd suffered, the way in which any treatment was supposed to work, and what I thought was the chance of success. He ran his body much as he ran his business. He wanted to be involved in every decision of importance, and he wanted decisions to be made only after all the relevant information had been collected and considered.

I decided to be wholly honest with him and, in a long, painful conversation, tried to break the appalling news as gently as I could. As I'd anticipated, I had to go through every detail of every test he'd had and discuss the relevance and implication of each finding.

He had one question to which I couldn't give an exact answer. How long did he have to live? It's a question which doctors in novels and films seem to have little trouble answering precisely. In real life, precision is impossible. Individual illnesses vary as much as do the individuals who suffer them, and – here lies the hope for us all – even the most deadly of diseases can regress in quite unexpected and unpredictable ways.

I explained this to my patient and in the end he got me to commit myself to the opinion that, if his illness ran the course it did in most other people, he would probably live for another eighteen months, maybe two years.

In fact, he survived for seventeen months, and he spent the first eight of those in a rigorous restructuring of the company for which he was responsible. Only when he died, seemingly unexpectedly, did people realise what he had been up to.

For years he had maintained his position as a buccaneer by surrounding himself with yes-men. In his few remaining months, he replaced them with better trained and more independently-minded executives. Then, just two months before he died, he resigned, having recruited a successor whom he reckoned would run the company in a different but no less successful way. The subsequent history of the company proved him right.

That was the most dramatic example I've encountered of the material implications of doctors' decisions on whether to tell patients the truth about their illnesses. The emotional consequences can be even greater. Yet while I and many of my colleagues believe that doctors should always be truthful with their patients, are there circumstances which would justify our being 'economical with the truth'?

The doctors' dilemma is not whether to lie or tell the truth but whether to tell every patient everything without being asked. There is one good reason for avoiding an absolute rule, particularly when the only information the doctor has to give is bad news: every patient does not want to hear it.

When the broadcaster Richard Dimbleby was being treated for the illness that eventually killed him, he often, after his treatment, had a drink with his doctors to discuss how things were going. But another broadcaster, Robert Robinson, has said emphatically that if he ever gets a nasty disease, he doesn't want anyone, including his doctor, to tell him anything about it. He would like doctors to get on with the business of treating the disease without burdening him with decisions about it.

The Dimbleby and the Robinson attitudes – when they are honestly proclaimed – are easy to deal with. But doctors have to cope with bewildering degrees of ambivalence that lie between.

Certainly, when I was a GP, I had patients, like the buccaneer, who thanked me for telling them the whole truth when the news was bad because it prevented them from making catastrophic decisions about their families or their businesses. But I also had the chilling experience of answering a patient's questions as honestly as I thought she wanted them answered and later having to face her accusation that I had destroyed any hope she had of enjoying what was left of her life.

The most we can ask of doctors is that, when it comes to judging what patients really want to know, they should, because of their training and experience, get it right more often than do others. Luckily, they don't have to rely only on their own experience. One of the most helpful contributions I have found to this debate came from a doctor who thought patients themselves might know best whether they should be told.

Some years ago a Kent chest physician, Dr John Spencer Jones, published the results of a study in which he had given an unusual option to some 200 patients who were being treated for an inevitably fatal form of cancer of the lung. He told them that, after tests for a number of named diseases including cancer, they would, if they asked, receive a truthful answer about the diagnosis. If they didn't want to know, all they needed to do was not ask.

Half the patients asked for the diagnosis and half deliberately did not. Later those who'd been given the full details were asked if they regretted their decision. Only one did. But after her death her husband said she eventually came to terms with the news and the knowledge had helped them both to understand her needs as she grew more ill.

The patients who didn't ask for the diagnosis explained that they just didn't want to know – though half of them later gave signs that they had guessed the nature of their illness, possibly because of the treatment they were having, possibly because their commonsense told them.

The survey also revealed the sort of ambivalence that makes rules difficult to draft. Just over 10 per cent of those who'd asked for the diagnosis later 'denied' that they'd been given it, talking as if their expectation of life was good though they'd been told it was not.

Dr Jones suggested that some of these probably did not want to know the truth in the first place but had been persuaded by their doctors' natural tendency to encourage hesitant patients. And some may have asked because they were confident that they were going to get good news, and when they got bad, suppressed it by denial.

Dr Jones's findings suggest that if doctors adopted an absolute policy – being wholly honest with all patients or with none – they could never suit more than half.

His findings also show quite clearly that the people who know best whether patients should be given all the details about their illness are the patients themselves.

Ideally you should let your family doctor know now what you'd like him to do if one day he has to decide how much to tell you. And ideally, if the decision has to be made, your doctor will not try to tell you any more than you ask for.

The Bottom Line

I suffer from a fatal disease and occasionally get a sharp reminder that the number of days I have left on this earth is rapidly diminishing.

Some of those reminders frighten me. Others make me sorry for myself. But every so often comes one that actually cheers me. The disease from which I suffer is a common one.

It's called mortality.

Though we're all aware that we move inevitably towards our deaths from the moment we're conceived, it's not a thought we want to keep at the front of our minds. Only the morbid would wish to make the contemplation of their deaths a dominant force in their lives.

Yet I suspect that many of us deny our mortality too energetically. We probably do it out of fear but a failure to acknowledge its existence can lead us into unreal decisions not just about personal or business affairs but about our health.

A year or two ago, on one of those golden days that come occasionally to Britain in November, I drove into the country to have lunch with a one-time patient who became a long-time friend. A year before he had had major surgery for the removal of a cancer and, the week we met, was due to revisit the hospital to hear what his surgeon wanted to do about a recurrence of the disease that had cast its shadow on an X-ray film.

But that wasn't what we talked about. We chatted about the things we always do: our work (he too is a writer who was once a scientist), news of our children, gossip about our friends, books we had read, plays and films we hoped to see.

I remember little of what he said but I shall never forget the mood of contentment that enwrapped him. He was so clearly at peace with the world that I commented on it. Only then did he tell me his recent medical history.

His treatment, he acknowledged, was a tribute to modern surgery. The right things had been done well and efficiently and he had been shown great kindness and consideration. But after modern technology had done its stuff he found himself cast upon a lonely shore.

Modern medicine didn't seem to have any suggestions as to how he could do what he most wanted to do, to 'fight' against the disease that seemed set on destroying him.

He searched energetically for the sort of help he wanted and found it only on the medical fringe and beyond. Because he is a scientist, he eventually rejected many of the mechanics of the 'fringe' treatments, but he has retained the spiritual qualities that the unorthodox practitioners encouraged him to develop.

During the thirty years that I have been a doctor my profession has acquired effective treatments for a host of diseases that we used to regard as incurable. This spectacular advance in medical knowledge has conditioned some doctors to treat mortality as an enemy to be fought on every front, rather than as an awkward ally which has occasionally to be appeased.

As a patient, I don't want doctors to capitulate in their 'fight against disease' but I would like them, as their technological weaponry grows more powerful, to remind themselves more often that their purpose is not to wage relentless war against mortality but to seek to improve the quality of the lives of all of us who suffer from it.

People talk these days about 'holistic medicine' – the treatment of the 'whole person' – as if it were a recent discovery. Yet the best medicine, or what I was brought up to think was the best medicine, has always been holistic, with doctors using their technical skills as wisely and considerately as they can to try to restore their patients into some sort of harmony with the world in which we all struggle to survive.

Forty years ago, doctors had more time to try to sustain the spirit of their patients while they also healed their bodies. These days they can become so preoccupied with the technology that they leave the spirit to fend for itself.

Their attitude may lead their patients also to accept that illness is a purely mechanical business so that they feel as lonely and abandoned as did my friend.

I re-learned from him that illness, particularly a serious illness, need not be a setback. It can be an opportunity to haul that suppressed awareness of mortality from the back of the mind and decide whether the things we think all-important as we sit in our 'executive offices' really do justify the place we give them in the hierarchy of our lives, an opportunity to remind ourselves of what it is that makes our life worth living, and of who it is who make our lives worthwhile.

One lesson I learned repeatedly from my patients when I was a family doctor was that, during serious illness, all the clichés can come true.

You really can discover who your best friends are and you really do have a chance to assess your life and change its direction, to discover that being healthy is not a matter of being mechanically sound in mind and body but of drawing strength from being part of a family, part of a community, a member of a species that can achieve harmonious though limited existence on this earth.

A patient once wrote to me: 'It's odd how illness made my life worth living. How awful it would have been if, instead of getting ill, I'd been hit by a bus and extinguished immediately, without ever learning what life really had to offer.' It's an observation worth considering by those whose lives are governed by the growing pile of paper in an 'in' tray.

Index